Promoting Inclusion Oral-Health

Promoting Inclusion Oral-Health

Social Interventions to Reduce Oral Health Inequities

Special Issue Editor

Ruth E. Freeman

MDPI • Basel • Beijing • Wuhan • Barcelona • Belgrade • Manchester • Tokyo • Cluj • Tianjin

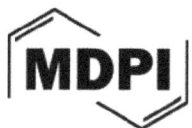

Special Issue Editor
Ruth E. Freeman
University of Dundee
UK

Editorial Office
MDPI
St. Alban-Anlage 66
4052 Basel, Switzerland

This is a reprint of articles from the Special Issue published online in the open access journal *Dentistry Journal* (ISSN 2304-6767) (available at: https://www.mdpi.com/journal/dentistry/special_issues/Reduce_Oral_Health_Disparities).

For citation purposes, cite each article independently as indicated on the article page online and as indicated below:

LastName, A.A.; LastName, B.B.; LastName, C.C. Article Title. *Journal Name* **Year**, *Article Number*, Page Range.

ISBN 978-3-03928-306-4 (Pbk)
ISBN 978-3-03928-307-1 (PDF)

© 2020 by the authors. Articles in this book are Open Access and distributed under the Creative Commons Attribution (CC BY) license, which allows users to download, copy and build upon published articles, as long as the author and publisher are properly credited, which ensures maximum dissemination and a wider impact of our publications.
The book as a whole is distributed by MDPI under the terms and conditions of the Creative Commons license CC BY-NC-ND.

Contents

About the Special Issue Editor vii

Preface to "Promoting Inclusion Oral-Health" ix

Ruth Freeman
Promoting Inclusion Oral Health: Social Interventions to Reduce Oral Health Inequities
Reprinted from: *Dentistry Journal* **2020**, *8*, , doi:10.3390/dj8010005 1

Laura Beaton, Emma Coles and Ruth Freeman
Homeless in Scotland: An Oral Health and Psychosocial Needs Assessment
Reprinted from: *Dentistry Journal* **2018**, *6*, , doi:10.3390/dj6040067 5

Ruth Freeman and Derek Richards
Factors Associated with Accessing Prison Dental Services in Scotland: A Cross-Sectional Study
Reprinted from: *Dentistry Journal* **2019**, *7*, , doi:10.3390/dj7010012 19

Laura Beaton, Isobel Anderson, Gerry Humphris, Andrea Rodriguez and Ruth Freeman
Implementing an Oral Health Intervention for People Experiencing Homelessness in Scotland:
A Participant Observation Study
Reprinted from: *Dentistry Journal* **2018**, *6*, , doi:10.3390/dj6040068 31

Andrea Rodriguez, Laura Beaton and Ruth Freeman
Strengthening Social Interactions and Constructing New Oral Health and Health Knowledge:
The Co-design, Implementation and Evaluation of A Pedagogical Workshop Program with and
for Homeless Young People
Reprinted from: *Dentistry Journal* **2019**, *7*, , doi:10.3390/dj7010011 45

Martijn Lambert
Dental Attendance in Undocumented Immigrants before and after the Implementation of
a Personal Assistance Program: A Cross-Sectional Observational Study
Reprinted from: *Dentistry Journal* **2018**, *6*, , doi:10.3390/dj6040073 61

Siyang Yuan
Evaluating an Oral Health Education Intervention in Chinese Undocumented Migrant Mothers
of Infants in Northern Ireland
Reprinted from: *Dentistry Journal* **2019**, *7*, , doi:10.3390/dj7010008 71

About the Special Issue Editor

Ruth Freeman a is Professor of Dental Public Health Research and an Honorary Consultant in Dental Public Health at the University of Dundee. She is the Director of the Oral Health and Health Research Programme, where she leads a multidisciplinary team researching inclusion oral health. She is Co-Director of the Dental Health Services Research Unit. She is a member of the British Psychoanalytic Council and a Fellow of the Faculty of Public Health, Royal College of Physicians (UK). She has published over 180 peer reviewed papers and 7 books in the joint areas of dental public health and behavioural sciences.

Preface to "Promoting Inclusion Oral-Health"

To advance our understanding of inclusion oral health and to address the impact of social exclusion on oral health, this book sets out to provide an argument for the need for social and community-based interventions, theoretically underpinned by pluralistic definitions of evidence-based practice and the radical discourse of health promotion for those experiencing exclusion. Using the definition and framework of inclusion oral health, these papers illustrate the requirement for mixed-methods research, the incorporation of experts by experience in the research process, and the need for co-design and co-produced interventions. The chapters in this edited book present various sources of evidence used to transform top-down into bottom-up community-based interventions for people experiencing homelessness, people in custody, and families residing in areas of high social deprivation. The first two chapters provide evidence of extreme oral health inequities in those experiencing exclusion, and the final four chapters report on the implementation and evaluation of social or community-based interventions. This collection of research papers will be of interest to all those wishing to reduce health inequities. This will be achieved by focusing on prevention, adopting a common risk factor agenda, and incorporating co-design and co-production elements into interventions, to tackle the oral health inequities felt by those most excluded in our societies.

Ruth E. Freeman
Special Issue Editor

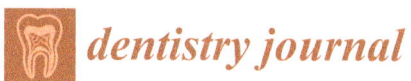

Editorial

Promoting Inclusion Oral Health: Social Interventions to Reduce Oral Health Inequities

Ruth Freeman

Dental Health Services Research Unit, Dundee Dental Hospital and School, University of Dundee, Dundee DD1 4HN, UK; r.e.freeman@dundee.ac.uk

Received: 13 December 2019; Accepted: 24 December 2019; Published: 7 January 2020

Abstract: To advance our understanding of inclusion oral health and to address the impact of social exclusion upon oral health, this group of papers sets out to provide an argument for the need for social and community-based interventions, theoretically underpinned by pluralistic definitions of evidence-based practice and the radical discourse of health promotion for those experiencing exclusion. Using the definition and framework of inclusion oral health, these papers illustrate the requirement for mixed-methods research, the incorporation of experts by experience in the research process, and the need for co-design and co-produced interventions. The papers in this Special Issue present various sources of evidence used to transform top-down into bottom-up community-based interventions for people experiencing homelessness, people in custody, and families residing in areas of high social deprivation. The first two papers provide the evidence for extreme oral health in those experiencing exclusion, and the final four papers report on the implementation and evaluation of social or community-based interventions. This collection of research papers will be of interest to all those wishing to reduce health inequities. This will be achieved by focusing on prevention, adopting a common risk factor agenda, and incorporating co-design and co-production elements into interventions, to tackle the oral health inequities felt by those most excluded in our societies.

Keywords: inclusion oral health; social exclusion; homelessness; prisons; undocumented migrants; social and community-based interventions

---

1. Introduction

The impact of people's health and disease was recognized in the first Global Burden of Disease report in 2010. Of the fifty nonfatal diseases identified world-wide, four of the diseases were dental caries in adults and children, chronic periodontitis, and edentulous [1]. Not only were dental diseases in the top fifty nonfatal illnesses, but dental caries in adults was tenth in the global burden of disease worldwide [2].

In 2018, Luchenski et al. studied the effect of disease on the most vulnerable populations. This work showed that, while a social gradient existed for the general population, for those experiencing social exclusion, a "so-called cliff-edge of inequality" occurred [3,4], resulting in "extreme health". To account for such health disparities, Luchenski and her colleagues proposed a definition for inclusion health as the means to "redress health and social inequities among the most vulnerable and marginalized in a community" [1].

It was to be another year before a coherent definition for inclusion oral health was available to address the oral health inequities of those "most vulnerable and marginalized" in our societies:

> *"Inclusion oral health is based on a theoretically engaged understanding of how social exclusion is produced and experienced, and how forms of exclusion and discrimination intersect to compound oral health outcomes. Inclusion oral health focuses on developing innovative inter-sectoral solutions to tackle the inequities of people enduring extreme oral health".* [5]

Underpinned by social exclusion, intersectionality, and othering theory, and the proposition that current dental systems acted as drivers for exclusion rather than inclusion, Freeman et al. [5] postulated a framework to promote oral health inclusion. This framework called for the following: the integration of health and social care policies to drive social justice and reduce prejudice and stigma; and the co-design and co-production of strategies formulated with and for people experiencing exclusion and the planning of "innovative, inter-sectorial services to promote inclusion" [5].

At the core of oral health inclusion were the research methods that provided a platform for experts by experience to contribute, together with the adoption of pluralistic definitions of evidence-based practice [6], to underpin oral health inclusion interventions [6–8]. This collection of papers gives the reader a cogent understanding of the role of evidence in the development of social or community-based interventions to promote inclusion oral health. These papers acknowledge the importance of mixed-method research; the role of experts by experience; and the adoption of a common risk factor agenda and the significance of focusing on prevention to tackle inequities experienced by those most excluded in our societies.

2. A Synopsis of the Special-Edition Papers

This special issue, entitled "Promoting Inclusion Oral-Health: Social Interventions to Reduce Oral Health Inequities", has attracted authors who are at the vanguard of inclusion oral health research. The examination of the predictors of oral health in people experiencing homelessness by Beaton et al. [9] and the influence of oral health impacts upon prisoners' decision to access dental care in prison [10] demonstrates the effect of extreme oral health upon those suffering social exclusion. Beaton et al. [9] and Freeman and Richards [10], therefore, provide the evidence for social interventions based on co-design and co-production strategies to promote oral health, within a common-risk-factor approach, for those experiencing social exclusion.

Returning to the framework of inclusion oral health [5], the papers by Beaton et al. [11] and Rodriguez et al. [12] on homelessness and Lambert [13] and Yuan [14] on undocumented migrants reflect the very essence of inclusion oral health. The requirement for mixed-methods research to include the voice of experts by experience in the research process is no clearer illustrated than in the papers of Beaton et al. [11] and Rodriguez et al. [12]. For Beaton et al. [11] it is the importance of working alliances between service users, health-care professionals, and the Third Sector that are necessary for the successful implementation of community-based programs to promote oral health. For Rodriguez et al. [12] it is the co-design and co-production of oral health and health promotion workshops, using Freire's [15] critical consciousness, that strengthens social interactions and knowledge transfer. By using oral health as a portal for knowledge development, the young people were able to voice their lived experiences of homelessness, and by doing so, they developed their life skills and their trust in others and strengthened their social interactions [12].

Acknowledging the need for "tuning into people's universe[s]" [15], Yuan [14] presents the case for cultural diversity for mother–infant community-based oral health improvement programs for undocumented migrants. The success of social support by using the vehicle of oral health intervention [16] is reported here by Yuan. Her work illustrates the importance of working with communities and advancing, "culturally appropriate approach[es] to improve undocumented migrant mothers' knowledge, attitudes, and self-reported behavior" when caring for their young child's oral health. The last paper is that by Lambert [13]. Examining the access to care for undocumented migrants, Lambert [13] takes the reader on a journey from extreme oral health to the acceptance of dental treatment. He convincingly shows that working within the system and training social workers as community oral health in an advocate role reduces missed appointments and provides a pathway for the integration of undocumented immigrants into "professional oral health care".

3. Conclusions

The papers in this special edition take the reader on a trajectory from extreme oral health to the co-design and co-production of interventions to tackle the oral health inequities suffered by those experiencing social exclusion. These papers will be of interested to all those who wish to confront oral health inequities, who wish to address "the cliff edge of inequality", and who wish to promote social justice through the advancement of inclusion oral health.

Funding: This research received no external funding.

Conflicts of Interest: The author declares no conflict of interest.

References

1. Vos, T.; Murray, J.L.; Lopez, A. Years Lived with Disability (YLDs) for 1,160 Sequelae of 289 Diseases and Injuries, 1990–2010: A Systematic Analysis for the Global Burden of Disease Study 2010. Available online: http://www.healthdata.org/research-article/years-lived-disability-ylds-1160-sequelae-289-diseases-and-injuries-1990%E2%80%932010 (accessed on 15 November 2019).
2. Marcenes, W.; Kassebaum, N.J.; Bernabe, E.; Flaxman, A.; Naghavi, M.; Lopez, A.; Murray, C.J. Global burden of oral conditions in 1990–2010: A systematic analysis. *J. Dent. Res.* **2013**, *92*, 592–597. [CrossRef] [PubMed]
3. Luchenski, S.; Psych, N.M.D.; Aldridge, R.W.; Hayward, A.; Story, A.; Perri, P.; Withers, J.; Clint, S.; Fitzpatrick, S.; Hewett, N. What works in inclusion health: Overview of effective interventions for marginalised and excluded populations? *Lancet* **2018**, *391*, 266–280. [CrossRef]
4. Aldridge, R.W.; Story, A.; Hwang, S.W. Morbidity and mortality in homeless individuals, prisoners, sex workers, and individuals with substance use disorders in high-income countries: A systematic review and meta-analysis. *Lancet* **2018**, *391*, 241–250. [CrossRef]
5. Freeman, R.; Doughty, J.; MacDonald, M.-E.; Muirhead, V. Inclusion oral health: Advancing a theoretical framework for policy, research and practice. *Community Dent. Oral Epidemiol.* **2019**. [CrossRef] [PubMed]
6. Holmes, D.; Murray, S.J.; Perron, A.; Rail, G. Deconstructing the evidence-based discourse in health sciences: Truth, power and fascism. *Int. J. Evid. Based Healthc.* **2006**, *4*, 180–186. [CrossRef] [PubMed]
7. Laverack, G.; Labonte, R. A planning framework for community empowerment goals within health promotion. *Health Policy Plan.* **2000**, *15*, 255–256. [CrossRef] [PubMed]
8. Freeman, R. Health promotion and the randomised controlled trial: A square peg in a round hole? *BMC Oral Health* **2009**. [CrossRef] [PubMed]
9. Beaton, L.; Rodriguez, A.; Freeman, R. Homeless in Scotland: An Oral Health and Psychosocial Needs Assessment. *Dent. J.* **2018**, *6*, 67. [CrossRef] [PubMed]
10. Freeman, R.; Richards, D. Factors Associated with Accessing Prison Dental Services in Scotland: A Cross-Sectional Study. *Dent. J.* **2019**, *7*, 12. [CrossRef] [PubMed]
11. Beaton, L.; Anderson, I.; Humphris, G.; Rodriguez, A.; Freeman, R. Implementing an Oral Health Intervention for People Experiencing Homelessness in Scotland: A Participant Observation Study. *Dent. J.* **2018**, *6*, 68. [CrossRef] [PubMed]
12. Rodriguez, A.; Beaton, L.; Freeman, R. Strengthening Social Interactions and Constructing New Oral Health and Health Knowledge: The Co-design, Implementation and Evaluation of a Pedagogical Workshop Program with and for Homeless Young People. *Dent. J.* **2019**, *7*, 11. [CrossRef] [PubMed]
13. Lambert, M. Dental Attendance in Undocumented Immigrants before and after the Implementation of a Personal Assistance Program: A Cross-Sectional Observational Study. *Dent. J.* **2018**, *6*, 73. [CrossRef] [PubMed]
14. Yuan, S. Evaluating an Oral Health Education Intervention in Chinese Undocumented Migrant Mothers of Infants in Northern Ireland. *Dent. J.* **2019**, *7*, 8. [CrossRef] [PubMed]

15. Freire, P. *Pedagogy of the Oppressed*; The Continuum International Publishing Group Inc.: London, UK, 1996.
16. Yuan, S.; Freeman, R. Can social support in the guise of an oral health education intervention promote mother–infant bonding in Chinese immigrant mothers and their infants? *Health Educ. J.* **2010**, *70*, 57–66. [CrossRef]

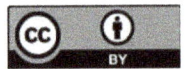

© 2020 by the author. Licensee MDPI, Basel, Switzerland. This article is an open access article distributed under the terms and conditions of the Creative Commons Attribution (CC BY) license (http://creativecommons.org/licenses/by/4.0/).

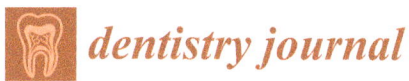

Article

Homeless in Scotland: An Oral Health and Psychosocial Needs Assessment

Laura Beaton [1,*], Emma Coles [2] and Ruth Freeman [1]

1. Dental Health Services Research Unit, University of Dundee, Dundee DD1 4HN, Scotland, UK; r.e.freeman@dundee.ac.uk
2. Nursing, Midwifery and Allied Health Professions Research Unit, University of Stirling, Stirling FK9 4NF, Scotland, UK; emma.coles@stir.ac.uk
* Correspondence: l.z.beaton@dundee.ac.uk; Tel.: +44-(0)1382740917

Received: 3 October 2018; Accepted: 13 November 2018; Published: 1 December 2018

Abstract: The aim of this research was to conduct an oral health and psychosocial needs assessment of a homeless population in Scotland to determine the levels of unmet need and provide recommendations for oral health improvement. A non-probability convenience sample of homeless people residing in seven Scottish Health Boards was collected. All consenting participants were asked to complete a questionnaire assessing their health and psychosocial needs, dental anxiety, and oral health-related quality of life. The participants' oral health was examined by a trained and calibrated dentist and dental nurse. Eight hundred and fifty-three homeless people consented to take part. Participants had a mean D_{3cv}MFT score of 16.9 (95% CI: 16.3, 17.6). Dental anxiety was high, with 20% scoring as dentally phobic. Respondents with higher dental anxiety were found to have significantly greater mean numbers of filled teeth than those with lower dental anxiety ($t = -2.9$, $p < 0.05$). Common oral health impacts were painful aching and discomfort while eating, experienced occasionally by 31% and 27% of the respondents, respectively. Fifty-eight percent of participants were found to have a depressive illness, and obvious decay experience was significantly higher among this section of participants ($t = -4.3$, $p < 0.05$). Homeless people in Scotland were found to be in need of a more accessible dental service than is currently available. An enhanced service should meet the oral health and psychosocial needs of this population to improve their oral health and quality of life.

Keywords: homeless persons; oral health; delivery of health care; dental health services

1. Introduction

In Scotland, between 2012 and 2013, 39,827 homelessness applications were made. Sixty-five percent of those making the applications were single people. The majority of applications (55%) were made by men. Thirty percent of homeless applications were from single households with children (i.e., one parent families). These were predominantly women (74%). While this, overall, represented a fall by some 13% in homelessness applications, the proportion of those considered as a priority, or frontline homeless, had risen by 5% between 2011 and 2013. This suggested that the number of those with an acute housing need had not fallen, but rather had increased [1]. While these statistics represent official homelessness figures, the true number of people experiencing homelessness in Scotland remains unknown, due to the concept of "hidden homelessness" and the inherent difficulties when defining homelessness. Therefore, the definition of homelessness used here was the European Typology of Homelessness, which defines homelessness in terms of accommodation [2]. Therefore, those who are roofless and those who are houseless (residing in insecure and/or inadequate accommodation) are characterized as experiencing homelessness.

Previous research has established that people experiencing homelessness have poor general and oral health. Hwang found that people experiencing homelessness had poor general health, a "high burden of illness" and "a greatly increased risk of death" [3] (pp. 232, 230). Regarding oral health, Daly et al. found that the oral health of people experiencing homelessness was poor, with a great need for restorative, oral hygiene, and periodontal treatment [4]. Figueiredo et al. confirmed that homeless populations had poor oral health, poor attendance, a reliance on emergency treatment, and unmet treatment needs [5].

The healthcare needs of homeless people in Scotland have long been recognised by the Scottish Government. In 2005 they produced the Health and Homelessness Standards, to ensure that National Health Service (NHS) Boards gave special consideration to improving the understanding, planning, and treatment of homeless people within their Board areas [6]. This was extended to the Action Plan for Improving Oral Health and Modernizing NHS Dental Services in Scotland (Dental Action Plan) in 2005. The Dental Action Plan recognised homeless people as a priority group, requiring tailored oral health care [7]. By 2012, the Scottish Government perceived that homeless people represented 'adults most in need', and in their Priority Group Strategy of 2012 [8] called for accessible oral health care facilities:

> 'Homeless people have a variety of challenges facing them. Many are affected by poor general health, low self-esteem and poorer than average dental health. They may have problems accessing facilities to carry out oral self-care and often have difficulty in accessing dental services.' (p. 2)

With the emphasis on accessible health care and preventive programs, the need to understand the oral health status together with homeless people's experiences of dental health care was seen as a first step in developing accessible services [9]. Therefore, the aim of this survey was to assess the oral health and psychosocial needs of homeless people across Scotland to allow recommendations for accessible dental health services to be made and to inform future oral health policy.

2. Materials and Methods

2.1. The Sample

A non-probability convenience sample of homeless people residing in seven National Health Services (NHS) Boards across Scotland was collected. In Scotland there are 14 NHS Boards, each representing a different geographical region, which provide primary and secondary level health care services to the population. In Scotland and in the United Kingdom, the NHS meets the needs of the population; is based on clinical need, not a person's ability to pay for treatment; and, it provides treatment that is free at the point of delivery [10]. The participating Scottish NHS Boards represented a mix of urban and rural localities (Figure 1).

Non-probability convenience sampling was used due to the transient nature of those experiencing homelessness, which can make them a difficult population to reach [11]. A number of different localities in each NHS Board were visited several times, in order to generate a snowball effect and thus maximize the number of participants consenting to take part (Table 1). Throughout the nine-month data collection period, homeless people were invited to take part and those consenting to participate were included.

Table 1. Details of data collection by participating National Health Services (NHS) Boards.

Board	Days/Times	Frequency	Staff	Venues
Board 1	Daytime only	1 session per week	1 dentist, 1 dental nurse, public health nurse administering questionnaire. Member of OHP Team to give opportunistic advice	Mainly hostels (may take place in drop-in center occasionally)
Board 2	Daytime only	1 session per week	1 dentist and 1 dental nurse	Hostels and the Salvation Army Drop-in Centre
Board 3	Daytime and occasional evenings	1 session per week	1 dentist and 1 dental nurse	Dental Clinic for Homeless People, Homeless Health Centre, indoor soup kitchen
Board 4	Daytime only	1 session per week	1 dentist, 1 dental nurse and an oral health coordinator	Hostels, residential units, day center, women's refuge, homeless van, plus the homeless service
Board 5	Wednesdays 6–9 pm	Once a week (visits to 2 establishments per night in one area)	Team of 3: dentist, dental nurse and administrator. Survey team consists of 4 dentists, 4 dental nurses and 1 senior HPO, working on a rota	Hostels and soup kitchens
Board 6	Daytime and occasional evenings	2 sessions per week	2 dentists and 2 dental nurses	Homeless Clinic, day centers, hostels, night shelter
Board 7	Daytime only	1 session per week	1 dentist, 1 dental nurse, 1 hygienist and/or public health nurse from homelessness health team	Hostels, day rooms

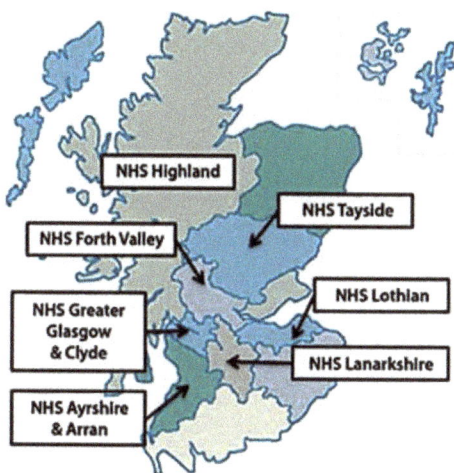

Figure 1. NHS Boards that participated in the Smile4life needs assessment (image reproduced from the Smile4life Report [12]).

2.2. Oral Health

1. Obvious Decay Experience

Obvious decay experience was assessed using the DMFT index in accordance with the National Dental Inspection Programme Basic Inspection procedures and the British Association for the Study of Community Dentistry guidelines, both of which state that this is "in accordance ... with international epidemiological conventions, thus allowing for comparisons to be made with other countries in Europe and beyond." [13] (p. 5). The dental status was recorded as obvious decay experience (D_{3cv}MFT), which recognised decay at the dentinal level (D_3), with visual cavitation (D_{3cv}) present. Obvious decay experience is the total D_{3cv}MFT, which is a sum of the decayed into dentine with cavitation (D_{3cv}), missing (M), and filled (F) teeth.

2. Assessment of Oral Hygiene Status: Plaque

Plaque scores were assessed using the Simplified Oral Hygiene Index (OHI-S) scale of debris present [14–16]. Plaque scores were assessed on six teeth, if present, with scores being given as follows: "0 = no debris or stain present; 1 = soft debris covering not more than 1/3 of the tooth surface, or presence of extrinsic stains without other debris, regardless of surface area covered; 2 = soft debris covering more than 1/3, but not more than two thirds, or exposed tooth surface; 3 = soft debris covering more than two thirds of exposed tooth surface" [12] (p. 35).

3. Oral Mucosa

An examination of the oral mucosa included the lips, buccal mucosa, tongue, floor of the mouth, palate and fauces. A score was allocated if a lesion was absent (0), lesion present and monitor (1), or requiring immediate referral (2).

An oral health survey collection form captured all of the information regarding the participants' obvious decay experience, plaque present, the number of standing teeth, and the incidence of oral mucosal lesions. The oral health examinations were conducted following completion of the questionnaire. The equipment used was a Daray light, disposable mirror, tweezers, and a WHO periodontal probe [17,18]. Other items, such as cotton wool pellets and rolls, were used where it was necessary to remove debris to visualize the oral structures.

The full examination was conducted under standardized conditions observing normal infection control protocols [19]. To ensure standardized data collection, prior to the survey commencement, the 11 dentists and 12 dental health professionals who were involved in the oral examination attended a training day where they were standardized using National Dental Inspection Programme (NDIP) training materials [20]. One month prior to this training day, the practitioners had been calibrated in accordance with NDIP.

2.3. The Questionnaire

The questionnaire consisted of four parts:

1. Demographic profile.

The questionnaire asked about the participants' age, gender, current and past living status, family status, previous occupation, and reason(s) for homelessness.

2. Medical history and health behaviors

This section examined the participants' medical history, including prescribed medication and health behaviors, such as alcohol, tobacco, and drug use.

3. Psycho-social status

Dental anxiety was assessed using the Modified Dental Anxiety Scale (MDAS) [21]. The MDAS consists of five questions assessing dental anxiety in relation to: waiting for dental treatment, drilling, scale and polish, and local anesthesia. Respondents rate their dental anxiety on a five-point scale, which ranges from not anxious (1) to extremely anxious (5). Possible scores range from 5 to 25, with scores over 19 indicating dental phobia. The normative value for a general practice patient population is 10.39 and the normative value for a UK general public population is 11.60 [22].

Oral Health Related-Quality of Life was assessed using the Oral Health Impact Profile (OHIP-14) [23]. This 14-item inventory was based on a hierarchy of impacts arising from oral disease, ranging in severity, and includes functional limitation (e.g., pronouncing words), physical pain (e.g., painful aching mouth), psychological discomfort (e.g., feeling self-conscious), physical disability (e.g., interrupted meals), psychological disability (e.g., feeling embarrassed), social disability (e.g., irritable with others), and handicap (e.g., life less satisfying). Respondents were asked how frequently they had experienced each of the 14 impacts, on a five-point Likert scale, with scores ranging from 0 (never) to 4 (very often).

Depression was measured using the valid and reliable Center for Epidemiological Studies Depression Scale (CES-D) [24]. The CES-D is a self-reported scale consisting of twenty items reflecting dimensions of depression, such as depressed mood, feelings of hopelessness, and interactions with others. The questions are answered on a four-point Likert scale and the respondents are asked to rate their experience of each item in the previous week, the responses ranged from rarely or none of the time (scoring 0) to most or all of the time (scoring 3). Total scores range from 0 to 60, with scores of 16 or over indicating depressed mood.

4. Previous dental experiences and dental health attitudes

The final part of the questionnaire inquired about the time and reason for the respondents' most recent dental attendance, as well as previous dental treatment experiences (e.g., fillings and extractions). Opinions about going to the dentist were also assessed, using nine attitudinal measures from the Adult Dental Health Survey [25], where responses were made on a four-point Likert scale, ranging from 'definitely feel like that' to 'don't feel like that'.

2.4. Administration of the Questionnaire

All dental health professionals and health practitioners who were involved in the administration of the questionnaire were provided with training tailored towards improving the understanding of the questionnaire prior to deployment, and how to engage with and assist participants with completion of the questionnaire items without influencing their responses. The participants were asked to complete the questionnaire prior to the oral examination. Many participants required help with completing the questionnaire due to poor eyesight and/or poor literacy skills.

2.5. Ethical Considerations

The National Research Ethics Service was contacted concerning the requirement for ethical approval. The Integrated Research Application System (IRAS) responded to state that ethical approval from an NRES was not required. This information was provided to each of the NHS Boards who obtained the relevant NHS Research and Development Management Approval. Ethical approval was obtained from the University of Dundee Research Ethics Committee (UREC 9005). Information sheets detailing each aspect of the survey, together with written consent forms, were provided to each participant. Homeless people were given an information sheet and a consent form. All participants were required to provide informed and written consent prior to taking part.

2.6. Statistical Analysis

The data was coded and entered onto a computer using SPSS version 19. Frequency distributions, *t*-tests, and regression analysis were performed on the data.

3. Results

3.1. Sample

A convenience sample of 853 people took part in the survey. There were 598 (70%) complete data sets, as some sections were not answered by all participants: for example, 45% did not give an occupation, 10% did not answer questions about their living status, and 36% did not give a reason for their homelessness. Eighty-five percent (726) of participants had an oral examination. The results shown below report on the complete data on each variable.

3.2. Oral Health Status

3.2.1. Obvious Decay Experience

The mean $D_{3cv}MFT$ was 16.9 (95% CI: 16.3, 17.6). The largest component was missing teeth (8.7 [95% CI: 8.1, 9.4]), with the number of missing teeth ranging from 0 to 32. The mean number of decayed teeth into dentine with visual cavitation was 4.5 (95% CI: 4.1, 4.9), with a range of 0 to 30. The mean number of filled teeth was 3.8 (95% CI: 3.5, 4.1). The number of filled teeth ranged from 0 to 25 teeth (Table 2). Female participants had significantly fewer mean numbers of filled teeth than men ($t = 2.22$, $p < 0.05$).

Table 2. Dental health status by age group.

Dental Health Status	Age Group (n)	Mean (95% CI)
Decay into dentine, cavitated and visual (D_{3cv})	16–24 (207)	4.05 (3.34, 4.77)
	25–34 (194)	6.24 (5.37, 7.11)
	35–44 (160)	4.14 (3.48, 4.79)
	45–54 (96)	3.16 (2.34, 3.97)
	55+ (51)	2.75 (1.47, 4.02)
Missing teeth	16–24 (207)	2.90 (2.36, 3.44)
	25–34 (194)	7.97 (6.89, 9.06)
	35–44 (160)	11.86 (10.42, 13.31)
	45–54 (96)	13.40 (11.52, 15.27)
	55+ (51)	16.55 (13.30, 19.80)
Filled teeth	16–24 (207)	3.09 (2.62, 3.56)
	25–34 (194)	3.60 (3.08, 4.11)
	35–44 (160)	4.02 (3.40, 4.63)
	45–54 (96)	5.07 (4.12, 6.02)
	55+ (51)	4.02 (2.64, 5.40)
Obvious decay experience ($D_{3cv}MFT$)	16–24 (207)	9.94 (8.92, 10.97)
	25–34 (194)	17.64 (16.53, 18.75)
	35–44 (160)	20.01 (18.73, 21.30)
	45–54 (96)	21.61 (20.18, 23.05)
	55+ (51)	23.31 (21.29, 25.34)
Standing teeth	16–24 (207)	26.45 (25.88, 27.02)
	25–34 (194)	22.43 (21.35, 23.50)
	35–44 (160)	18.51 (17.10, 19.91)
	45–54 (96)	17.03 (15.09, 18.97)
	55+ (51)	13.43 (10.37, 16.49)

3.2.2. Assessment of Oral Hygiene Status: Plaque

The total mean plaque score for the sample population was 1.08 (95% CI: 1.01, 1.15). The mean plaque score for the upper teeth was 1.06 (95% CI: 0.99, 1.13) and for the lower teeth 1.10 (95% CI: 1.04, 1.16).

3.2.3. Oral Mucosa

The oral examination assessed the six areas of the mouth and throat that are listed in the methods section. The most frequent location of a suspicious lesion was in the buccal mucosa (4%), followed by the lips (3%), palate (2%), tongue (1%), floor of the mouth (0.3%), and throat (0.2%). Overall, 61 participants (9%) had one suspicious oral mucosal lesion and six participants had two.

3.2.4. Edentulousness

Forty-six (6%) of the 726 participants who underwent the oral examination had no natural teeth.

3.3. Demographic Profile

Seventy-four percent (629) of the participants were male, with ages ranging from 16 to 78. The mean age was 33.9 (95% CI: 33.1, 34.7). Age was divided into five age groups; with 207 participants being aged between 16–24 years; 194 being aged between 25–34 years; 160 being aged between 35–44 years; 160 being aged between 45–54 years; and, 51 being aged 55 years and over. Of those who answered the question on family type (805), 77% reported that they were single, with 13% having a partner and 4% and 6% being part of a one-parent family and two-parent family, respectively.

Six hundred and ninety-four participants (81%) answered the "Living status" section, with 83 participants not responding and 76 people giving more than one answer. From those that did respond, 560 were classed as "houseless" (73%) and 46 were "roofless" (6%).

Occupation/previous occupation was taken as an indicator of socio-economic position [26]. Of those that did provide information about their occupation, 25% worked in skilled trade occupations and 22% worked in unskilled occupations. Forty-five percent of participants did not provide details about their current or previous occupation and were assumed to be "economically inactive" [12] (p. 41).

3.4. Reasons for Becoming Homeless

Of the 542 participants that provided a reason for homelessness, the most frequent reason was family breakdown (22%), followed by imprisonment (11%), alcohol (9%), domestic violence (8%), drug misuse (7%), financial difficulties (6%), mental or physical ill-health (4%), relocation (3%), and unemployment (2%).

3.5. Medical History and Health Behaviors

Of those that completed the medical history (787), 54% reported that they were currently receiving medical treatment. Twenty-two percent reported having chest diseases; 13% reported suffering from hypertension, 7% had epilepsy, 7% had heart disease, and 3% had diabetes. Eleven percent of respondents stated that they were HIV-positive or Hepatitis C-positive (11%).

Sixty-three percent (496) of those that completed the medical history also stated that they were taking prescribed medication, and 472 of the 496 provided the name and type of medication that they were prescribed. The most commonly mentioned prescribed medications were psychotrophic drugs (i.e., antidepressants (32%), anxiolytics (20%), and anti-psychotics (11%)) and methadone (32%).

When asked about alcohol and tobacco consumption, 29% (240) of respondents stated that they drank alcohol "most days" and 85% (702) reported that they smoked tobacco.

Regarding drug use, 68% of respondents reported that they had a history of street drug use. Of the 68%, 236 (29%) reported that they were currently using street drugs and of the 236, 191 stated that they were currently injecting drug users. With regard to age, significantly lower proportions of those aged 55 years and over as compared with the other lower age groups that stated that they had ever used drugs ($X2[4] = 121.60$, $p < 0.001$), were currently using drugs ($X2[4] = 37.12$, $p < 0.001$) or were injecting drug users ($X2[4] = 51.34$, $p < 0.001$). Equivalent proportions of male (68%) and female (66%) respondents reported to have used street drugs; currently using drugs (male: 30%; female 26%) and being injecting drug users (male 23%; female 29%).

3.6. Dental Anxiety Status

Of the 799 participants who completed the MDAS, the mean score for dental anxiety was 12.1 (95% CI: 11.6, 12.6). Twenty percent (170) scored over 19, which indicates that they were dentally phobic. Women as compared to men had significantly higher mean scores for dental anxiety ($t = 5.85$, $p < 0.001$). This sample was split into higher and lower dental anxiety—respondents who scored 12 or less (324) were categorized as having lower dental anxiety, while those that scored 13 or higher (475) were deemed to have high dental anxiety. The respondents with higher dental anxiety had a significantly higher mean number of filled teeth when compared to the lower dental anxiety group, whereas those with lower dental anxiety had significantly higher mean numbers of decayed teeth as compared to those with higher anxiety. There were no other significant differences (Table 3).

Table 3. Comparison of low and high dental anxiety status with oral health status.

Oral Health Status	Lower Dental Anxiety Status (n = 271) Mean (95% CI)	Higher Dental Anxiety Status (n = 414) Mean (95% CI)	t	p
$D_{3cv}MFT$	17.2 (16.1, 18.3)	16.6 (15.8, 17.5)	0.7	0.46
Decayed teeth	6.0 (5.4, 6.8)	3.5 (3.1, 3.9)	5.9	<0.05
Missing teeth	8.0 (7.1, 9.0)	9.0 (8.1, 9.9)	−1.4	0.17
Filled teeth	3.2 (2.8, 3.7)	4.1 (3.7, 4.5)	−2.9	<0.05

3.7. Oral Health Related Quality of Life

Seven-hundred and thirty-two participants completed the OHIP-14 section of the questionnaire. The mean score for oral health impacts was 17.1 (95% CI: 16.0, 18.1). Women experienced significantly more oral health impacts when compared to men ($t = 2.39$, $p < 0.05$). The oral health impacts that were reported by participants are shown in Figure 2. Twenty-five percent (200) of participants felt self-conscious and 23% (190) felt embarrassed very often about the appearance of their mouth and teeth. The oral health impact 'painful aching' was experienced occasionally by 31% of the respondents; fairly often by 17%; and, very often by 12%. Twenty-seven percent reported that they occasionally felt discomfort while eating.

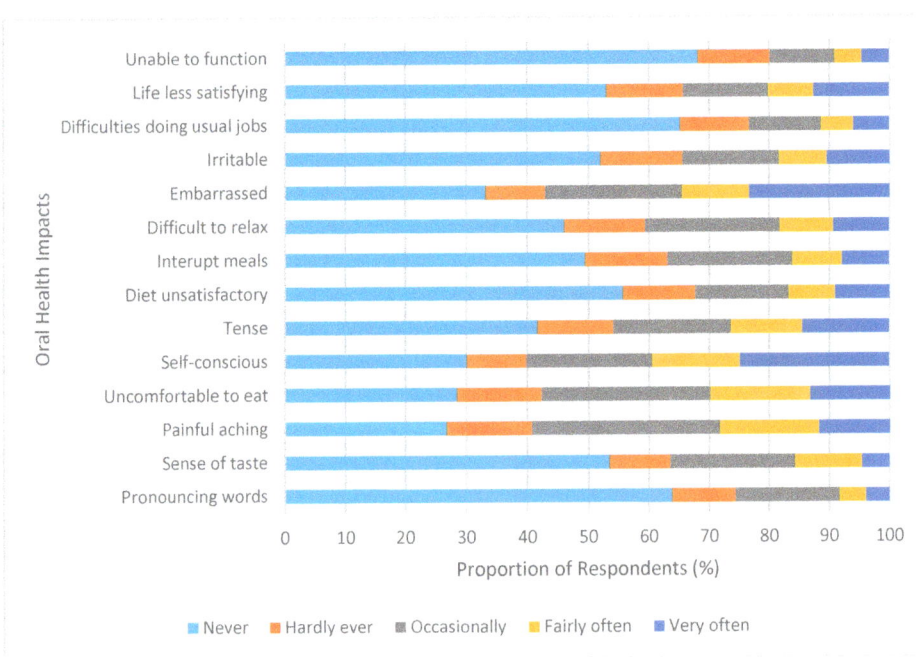

Figure 2. Frequency of oral health impacts.

The sample was divided into lower and higher oral health-related quality of life impact groups using a median split—those scoring 14 or less were categorized as experiencing lower impacts, while those scoring 15 or over experienced higher impacts. Significant differences were found between lower and higher oral health impact experiences for decayed, missing, and filled teeth, as well as overall obvious decay experience (Table 4). The mean numbers of decayed and missing teeth were significantly higher for those with higher oral health impact experience, while the mean number of filled teeth was significantly higher for the lower impact group. The mean $D_{3cv}MFT$ was significantly higher for those experiencing higher, rather than lower, oral health impacts.

Table 4. Comparison of low and high oral impact experience with obvious decay experience.

Oral Health Status	Low Oral Health Impact Experience (n = 338) Mean (95% CI)	High Oral Health Impact Experience (n = 298) Mean (95% CI)	t	p
$D_{3cv}MFT$	14.6 (13.7, 15.7)	19.2 (18.2, 20.0)	−6.5	<0.05
Decayed teeth	2.8 (2.4, 3.2)	6.4 (5.7, 7.1)	−8.8	<0.05
Missing teeth	7.8 (6.8, 8.8)	9.5 (8.6, 10.5)	−2.4	<0.05
Filled teeth	4.0 (3.6, 4.5)	3.3 (2.9, 3.8)	2.2	<0.05

3.8. Depression

Of the 562 participants who completed the CES-D, 58% (328) scored at least 16, which indicates that they were suffering from a depressive illness. The mean score for depression was 21.7 (95% CI: 20.5, 22.8). Women had significantly higher mean depression scores (t = 3.25, p = 0.001) when compared to men, with the mean score for women being 24.8 (95% CI: 22.6, 27.0) and for men 20.5 (95% CI: 19.2, 21.9). The sample was divided into "not depressed" (scores < 16) and "depressed" (scores > 16). Depressed participants had significantly higher mean numbers of decayed teeth and $D_{3cv}MFT$ as compared to participants who were not depressed (Table 5). Regression analysis was used to predict the effect of age, gender, and depression upon obvious decay experience. Age and depression significantly predicted obvious decay experience and explained 25% of the variance in the relationship $F[2, 503] = 55.95, p < 0.001$ (Table 6).

Table 5. Comparison of obvious decay experience with depression.

Oral Health Status	Not Depressed (n = 222) Mean (95% CI)	Depressed (n = 297) Mean (95% CI)	t	p
$D_{3cv}MFT$	14.0 (12.8, 15.3)	17.4 (16.5, 18.3)	−4.3	<0.05
Decayed teeth	3.8 (3.1, 4.4)	5.5 (4.8, 6.2)	−3.7	<0.05
Missing teeth	7.0 (5.9, 8.2)	8.2 (7.2, 9.1)	−1.5	0.13
Filled teeth	3.3 (2.8, 3.8)	3.7 (3.3, 4.2)	−1.3	0.19

Table 6. The effect of age, gender and depression as predictors of obvious decay experience.

Independent Variables	B	SE	t	p
Gender	−0.12	0.79	−0.14	0.89
Age	3.29	0.28	11.84	<0.001
Depression	0.09	0.02	3.73	<0.001
$F[2, 503] = 55.95, p < 0.001: R^2 = 0.25$.				

3.9. Previous Dental Experiences and Dental Health Attitudes

3.9.1. Dental Attendance

Three-hundred and forty-six participants reported that they had been to the dentist in the last year, with 31% of respondents reporting that they were registered with a dentist (at the time of data collection). From those who gave a reason for their last dental visit, 68% reported that they attended due to "trouble with teeth" and 21% attended for a check-up.

3.9.2. Previous Dental Treatment

The most frequently cited previous treatment experience was receiving an injection in the gum (92%), followed by fillings (89%) and extractions (81%). The least common treatment experience was bridgework, with only 12% of respondents undergoing this treatment.

3.9.3. Dental Health Attitudes

When questioned about dental health attitudes, the number of respondents varied from 797 to 809. The most common attitude was "I'd like to be able to drop in at the dentist without an appointment", with 62% of participants stating that they "definitely" felt like that. This was followed by "I'd like to know more about what the dentist is going to do and why" (37%).

4. Discussion

Policies from the Scottish Government over the last decade [6–8] have sought to improve access and support for homeless people accessing dental treatment. The 2005 Health and Homelessness Standards stated that "there are a wide range of health problems which are more prevalent amongst homeless people than the wider population ... chronic diseases ... infectious diseases." [6] (p. 12). There was no mention, however, of oral health in this document. This changed with the Dental Action Plan [7], and the importance of oral health status was reinforced by the National Oral Health Improvement Strategy for Priority Groups, which made the oral health of homeless people a priority [8]. Therefore, to inform policy and improve accessible services, there was a need to conduct a survey to assess the oral health status and psychosocial needs of people that were affected by homelessness in Scotland.

The 853 homeless people who took part in this needs assessment reflected the profile of similar homeless populations elsewhere, as well as the composition of the Scottish homeless population, particularly in terms of age and gender distribution, with the majority of participants being male, with a mean age of 33.9 [1,27]. The majority of participants were "houseless", instead of "roofless", meaning that they were currently living in a hostel, temporary accommodation, or similar, and were not sleeping rough. A wide range of reasons were given for how the participants had originally become homeless. The most common reason given was family breakdown, which was also found to be a frequent reason for homelessness in North and West Belfast [27], along with substance misuse (alcohol and drug use).

The prevalence of smoking in this sample of participants was high, with 85% reporting that they smoked tobacco. This high percentage is surprising when it is contrasted with the comparatively low 23% of adults in Scotland that indicated they were smokers in the 2013 Scottish Household Survey [28]. Regarding alcohol consumption, the participants in this sample drank more than the general Scottish population: 12% of adults reported in the 2012 Scottish Health Survey that they drank more than five days in a week, as compared to the 29% of this sample who reported drinking most days [29]. A high smoking rate, coupled with regular excessive alcohol consumption places this population at a high risk of developing oral cancer [6,29]. In this sample, 61 participants were found to have suspicious oral mucosal lesions. Five of these required referral to secondary services.

Similarly, the high number of participants prescribed anti-depressants and methadone is not reflected in the general population. Reports from Information Services Division (ISD) Scotland show that approximately 11.3% of the Scottish population were prescribed some form of anti-depressant in 2010/11, while 122 people per 1000 population were prescribed methadone [30,31].

High levels of obvious decay experience, as well as the prevalence of edentulousness, indicates that homeless people in Scotland were not accessing or receiving the necessary level of treatment. The obvious decay experience of the population in this sample is poorer than that of the Scottish population as a whole, with a higher average number of missing and decayed teeth, and lower numbers of filled teeth [25]. However, the Scotland Health Survey (2012 edition) found that in 2012 10% of adults had no natural teeth, but in this sample population, only 6% of participants were edentulous [32].

The homeless population in this sample were found to have high levels of dental anxiety: 20% scored over 19 on the MDAS and were therefore classed as having high dental anxiety, or dental phobia. The proportion of the general UK population scoring above this cut-off is 11% [22]. It is possible that the dental anxiety in this population had developed due to negative past experiences of dental treatment, as those with high dental anxiety also had significantly more filled teeth as compared to those with low dental anxiety. This theory is strengthened by the finding that the low dental anxiety group had significantly more decayed teeth, indicating a poor history of dental attendance and therefore limited opportunity to have a negative dental experience—indeed, only one-third of participants were registered with a dentist at the time the questionnaire was administered.

Higher prevalence of obvious decay experience has clear implications for oral health-related quality of life, as decayed or decaying teeth can cause discomfort or pain, which in turn can have serious impacts on day-to-day functioning. Indeed, significant differences were found between high and low oral health impacts and $D_{3cv}MFT$, with higher incidences of missing and decayed teeth associated with higher oral health impact. In the Adult Dental Health Survey, which studied the oral health of the United Kingdom, the most common impacts were categorized as physical pain, psychological discomfort, and psychological disability [25]. The findings from this assessment represented a similar result, with painful aching and discomfort (physical pain) being the most common impacts, followed by self-consciousness (psychological discomfort) and embarrassment (psychological disability). It is worth noting, however, that, when compared to the general population in Scotland, higher proportions of respondents in this survey experienced psychological discomfort and psychological disability regarding their teeth, mouth, and dentures [12].

Previous research has highlighted that depression among homeless people can be as high as up to four times the rate of the general population [33]. In this sample, the mean score for women was 24.8 and for men 20.5, which is considerably higher than that of the general population in the United Kingdom (14.2 for women and 13.4 for men), although, in accordance with the general UK population norms, women's scores were higher than men's [34]. Moreover, a significant relationship was shown between obvious decay experience with age and depression, suggesting that depression had an important influence upon oral health status. This is supported by the work of Coles et al., which showed that 19% of the depression could be explained by decayed and missing teeth in a homelessness population [35]. The implications of such findings are important, since they suggest the need for inclusion of oral health and multidisciplinary working between health, social care, and oral health services.

This assessment was affected by some limitations. First, participants were gathered from the more urban areas of Scotland, which allowed greater access to this group of participants, but perhaps did not allow for the collection of information from the more rural population, which may have its own unique barriers to dental treatment. Also, the response rate was particularly poor for some sections of the questionnaire, specifically "occupation" and "reasons for homelessness". While participants may have left the "occupation" section blank because they were currently unemployed, participants may have left other sections blank because of the sensitive and potentially emotive nature of some of the questions.

In conclusion, the stressful and often apparent chaotic lifestyle of the homeless population has serious consequences for the general health and wellbeing of this group, and, more specifically, their oral health. When compared to the Scottish and UK general populations, the participants in this needs assessment had poorer oral and psychosocial health. Depression and dental anxiety were found to be more prevalent in this sample than in the general population. Similarly, smoking and alcohol consumption levels were higher than national averages, as were the number of people prescribed anti-depressants and methadone.

These findings highlight that the oral health and psychosocial needs of the homeless population of Scotland are markedly different from those of the general population. As such, it is necessary to adopt a "bottom-up" approach, whereby people experiencing homelessness are encouraged to share their needs and concerns regarding oral health to help shape future oral health improvement interventions. A tailored approach that takes into account the psychosocial needs of the homeless population, not just their oral health, is therefore recommended as a method of improving the oral health and wellbeing of people affected by homelessness in Scotland. Indeed, following the needs assessment, an intervention, called Smile4life, was developed, alongside a Guide for Trainers resource, to help health and social care practitioners address the oral health needs of people experiencing homelessness [36]. The Smile4life Guide for Trainers intervention was recommended in Government strategy [8] as the approach to be taken by dental health and social care professionals to improve the oral health of people experiencing homelessness.

The provision of dental services should also be reconsidered. The findings from this study suggest that there is a reliance on emergency treatment, as indicated by the low prevalence of restored teeth. While that is perhaps appropriate for those in immediate need, there should also be a focus on providing preventive treatment alongside restorations for individuals that are able to access routine dental care. A comprehensive dental service that meets the differing needs of the homeless population should allow better access to services, which, in turn, should improve the oral health of this population group.

Author Contributions: Conceptualization, R.F.; Formal analysis, L.B.; Funding acquisition, R.F.; Investigation, E.C. and R.F.; Methodology, E.C. and R.F.; Supervision, R.F.; Visualization, L.B.; Writing—original draft, L.B.; Writing—review & editing, L.B., E.C. and R.F.

Funding: The Smile4life Programme was funded by the Scottish Government and National Health Service Boards, grant number: 121.80.4497.

Acknowledgments: The authors wish to thank the Scottish Government Health Department and the NHS Boards involved in the collection of data (award number 121.804497), and the Smile4life steering group for its valued contributions.

Conflicts of Interest: The authors declare no conflict of interest.

References

1. Scottish Government. *Operation of the Homeless Persons Legislation 2012–13*; Scottish Government: Edinburgh, Scotland, 2013.
2. Edgar, B.; Meert, H. *Fourth Review of Statistics on Homelessness in Europe*; European Observatory on Homelessness: Brussels, Belgium, 2005.
3. Hwang, S.W. Homelessness and health. *CMAJ* **2001**, *164*, 229–233. [PubMed]
4. Daly, B.; Newton, T.; Batchelor, P.; Jones, K. Oral health care needs and Oral Health-Related Quality of Life (OHIP-14) in homeless people. *Community Dent. Oral Epidemiol.* **2010**, *38*, 136–144. [CrossRef] [PubMed]
5. Hwang, S.W.; Quiñonez, C. Dental health of homeless adults in Toronto, Canada. *J. Public Health Dent.* **2013**, *73*, 74–78.
6. Scottish Executive. *Health and Homelessness Standards*; Scottish Executive: Edinburgh, Scotland, 2005.
7. Scottish Executive. *An Action Plan for Improving Oral Health and Modernising NHS Dental Services in Scotland*; Scottish Executive: Edinburgh, Scotland, 2005.
8. Scottish Government. *National Oral Health Improvement Strategy for Priority Groups: Frail Older People, People with Special Care Needs and Those Who are Homeless*; Scottish Government: Edinburgh, Scotland, 2005.
9. British Dental Association. *Dental Care for Homeless People, BDA Policy Discussion Paper*; British Dental Association: London, UK, 2004.
10. NHS Principles and Values. Available online: https://www.nhs.uk/using-the-nhs/about-the-nhs/principles-and-values/ (accessed on 24 October 2018).
11. Hulley, S.B.; Cummings, S.R.; Browner, W.S.; Grady, D.G.; Newman, T.B. *Designing Clinical Research*, 4th ed.; Lippincott Williams & Wilkins: Philadelphia, PA, USA, 2013.
12. Coles, E.; Edwards, M.; Elliot, G.; Freeman, R.; Heffernan, A.; Moore, A. *Smile4life: The Oral Health of Homeless People in Scotland*; University of Dundee: Dundee, Scotland, 2011.

13. Macpherson, L.M.D.; Conway, D.I.; McMahon, A.D.; Watling, C.; Mahmoud, A.; O'Keefe, E.J.; Trainer, A.; White, V. *National Dental Inspection Programme (NDIP) 2018: Report of the 2018 Detailed Inspection Programme of Primary 1 Children and the Basic Inspection of Primary 1 and Primary 7 Children*; ISD Scotland: Edinburgh, Scotland, 2018.
14. Löe, H. The gingival index, the plaque index and the retention index systems. *J. Periodontol.* **1967**, *38*, 610–616. [CrossRef]
15. Reddy, S. *Essentials of Clinical Periodontology and Periodontics*, 2nd ed.; Jaypee Brothers: New Delhi, India, 2008.
16. Crippen, D.J.; Wood, A.F.; Chambers, D.W. Initial plaque score as an indicator of patient appointment compliance. *J. Calif. Dent. Assoc.* **2003**, *31*, 621–625. [PubMed]
17. Mullen, J.; McGaffin, J.; Farvardin, N.; Brightman, S.; Haire, C.; Freeman, R. Caries status in 16 year-olds with varying exposure to water fluoridation in Ireland. *Community Dent. Health* **2012**, *29*, 293–296. [PubMed]
18. Mitropoulos, C.; Pitts, N.B.; Deery, C. *British Association for the Study of Community Dentistry Criteria for the Standardised Assessment of Dental Health (1992/93)*; University of Dundee: Dundee, Scotland, 1992.
19. Scottish Dental Clinical Effectiveness Programme. *Decontamination into Practice: Dental Clinical Guidance*; Scottish Dental Clinical Effectiveness Programme: Dundee, Scotland, 2011.
20. Macpherson, L.M.D.; Ball, G.; Conway, D.I.; Edwards, M.; Goold, S.; O'Hagan, P.; McMahon, A.D.; O'Keefe, E.J.; Pitts, N.B. *Report of the 2012 Detailed National Dental Inspection Programme of Primary 1 Children and the Basic Inspection of Primary 1 and Primary 7 Children*; ISD Scotland: Edinburgh, Scotland, 2012.
21. Humphris, G.M.; Morrison, T.; Lindsay, S.J.E. The modified dental anxiety scale: Validation and United Kingdom norms. *Community Dent. Health* **1995**, *12*, 43–150.
22. Humphris, G.M.; Dyer, T.A.; Robinson, P.G. The modified dental anxiety scale: UK general public population norms in 2008 with further psychometrics and effects of age. *BMC Oral Health* **2009**, *9*, 20. [CrossRef] [PubMed]
23. Locker, D. Measuring oral health: A conceptual framework. *Community Dent. Health* **1988**, *5*, 5–13.
24. Radloff, L.S. The CES-D Scale: A self-report depression scale for research in the general population. *Appl. Psychol. Meas.* **1977**, *1*, 385–401. [CrossRef]
25. Kelly, M.; Steele, J.; Nuttall, N.; Bradnock, G.; Morris, J.; Nunn, J.; Pine, C.; Pitt, N.; Treasure, E.; White, D. *Adult Dental Health Survey: Oral health in the United Kingdom 1998*; The Stationery Office: London, UK, 2000.
26. Office for National Statistics. *Standard Occupational Classification 2000*; The Stationary Office: London, UK, 2000.
27. Collins, J.; Freeman, R. Homeless in North and West Belfast: An oral health needs assessment. *Br. Dent. J.* **2007**, *202*, E31. [CrossRef] [PubMed]
28. Scottish Government. *Scottish Household Survey Annual Report—Scotland's People*; Scottish Government: Edinburgh, Scotland, 2013.
29. Health Development Agency. *Homelessness, Smoking and Health*; Health Development Agency: London, UK, 2004.
30. ISD Scotland. *Prescribing and Medicine: Medicines Used in Mental Health*; ISD Scotland: Edinburgh, Scotland, 2011.
31. ISD Scotland. *Drug Misuse Statistics Scotland 2011*; ISD Scotland: Edinburgh, Scotland, 2012.
32. Scottish Government. *The Scottish Health Survey*, 2012 ed.; Scottish Government: Edinburgh, Scotland, 2012.
33. Wong, Y.-L.I. Measurement properties of the Center for Epidemiologic Studies—Depression Scale in a Homeless Population. *Psychol. Assess.* **2000**, *12*, 69–76. [CrossRef] [PubMed]
34. Van de Velde, S.; Bracke, P.; Levecque, K.; Meuleman, B. Gender differences in depression in 25 European countries after eliminating measurement bias in the CES-D 8. *Sci. Soc. Res.* **2010**, *39*, 396–404. [CrossRef]
35. Coles, E.; Chan, K.; Collins, J.; Humphris, G.M.; Richards, D.; Williams, B.; Freeman, R. Decayed and missing teeth and oral-health-related factors: Predicting depression in homeless people. *J. Psychosom. Res.* **2011**, *71*, 108–112. [CrossRef] [PubMed]
36. Freeman, R.; Coles, E.; Watt, C.; Edwards, M.; Jones, C. *Smile4life Guide for Trainers: Better Oral Care for Homeless People*; NHS Health Scotland: Edinburgh, Scotland, 2012.

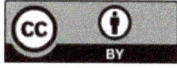

© 2018 by the authors. Licensee MDPI, Basel, Switzerland. This article is an open access article distributed under the terms and conditions of the Creative Commons Attribution (CC BY) license (http://creativecommons.org/licenses/by/4.0/).

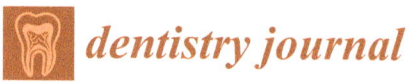

Article

Factors Associated with Accessing Prison Dental Services in Scotland: A Cross-Sectional Study

Ruth Freeman [1,2,*] and Derek Richards [3,4]

1. Dental Health Services Research Unit, University of Dundee, Dundee DD1 4HN, UK
2. Public Health, NHS Tayside, Dundee, DD2 1UB, UK
3. Centre for Evidence-based Dentistry, DHSRU, University of Dundee, Dundee DD1 4HN, UK; derek.richards@nhs.net
4. Dental Public Health South East Scotland, NHS Forth Valley, Stirling FK9 4SW, UK
* Corresponding author: r.e.freeman@dundee.ac.uk

Received: 12 December 2018; Accepted: 29 January 2019; Published: 1 February 2019

Abstract: Background: Prisoners have poorer dental health than non-prison populations. It is known that the prison environment can promote health and thus, policies, including access to dental care, are in place to promote health during imprisonment. **Aim:** Our aim was to conduct an oral health and psychosocial needs survey to identify the factors associated with accessing prison dental services in Scotland. **Methods:** A convenience sample of offenders from a male maximum security prison, a women's prison, and a young offenders' institution was gathered. A questionnaire examined the demography, prison experience, dental anxiety, oral health-related quality of life, and reported attendance of dental services. A dental examination was conducted using the International Caries Detection and Assessment System to diagnose obvious decay. A hierarchical logistic regression analysis was performed. **Results:** 342 prisoners participated. When missing data were excluded, the final sample was 259. The regression analysis showed the following: Model 1 characterized the offenders by demography and prison experience, explaining 19% of the variance. Model 2 showed that an offender was 36% more likely to attend dental services for every unit change in the 5-point ranking scale of 'feeling irritable with people because of teeth, mouth, or dentures', explaining an additional 7% of the variance. Model 3 explained 35% of the variance, (i.e., an additional 9%) and was adopted as the final model to characterize offenders who access dental services when in prison. An offender who reported accessing prison dental services was 3.28 times more likely to be male. For each increase in the year of an offender's age, the offender was 5% more likely to access prison dental services. An 11% greater chance of accessing prison dental services for every experience of remand was also found. An offender was 32% more likely to access prison dental services for each increased level of irritability, and there was a 2 times higher likelihood of emergency dental services' attendance. There was a 19% lower chance of accessing prison dental services for each additional tooth affected by decay and a 13% greater chance of accessing prison dental services for each unit increase in missing teeth. **Conclusions:** In conclusion, this investigation identified factors associated with access to prison dental services in Scotland. The role of accessibility factors, such as the oral health impact of irritability, appeared to increase perceptions of dental need and promote dental services' attendance.

Keywords: prison; accessible dental services; oral health-related quality of life; obvious decay

1. Background

Prisoners have greater numbers of decayed and missing teeth but fewer filled teeth when compared with the non-prison population [1–7]. While lifestyle issues prior to imprisonment are important, the prison environment with its routines and structures can promote oral health while also having the potential to exacerbate unhealthy behaviors [2,5,6]. Consequently, the concept of the health-promoting prison has moved to center stage, ensuring that policies have been put in place to promote health within the prison environment [8–10]. The promotion of oral health, for instance, is a central strand of the World Health Organization's European policy for offenders and ex-offenders. Attendance of dental care services has been linked to improved self-care and quality of life for offenders and ex-offenders [8–10].

Current research reports that people in prison, even when they have toothache [1–3,5–7], experience difficulties when trying to access dental services [5]. It would seem appropriate, therefore, to investigate the background factors related to the utilization of prison dental services. The difficulties people in prison encounter when accessing dental services are stated to be associated with poor literacy, poor health literacy, dental fear, and low perception of need [5,11–15]. These so-called 'patient factors' are reflected in Cohen's [16] accessibility framework. However, the observations that 23% of offenders reported that they had a pattern of regular dental attendance for examination and routine dental treatment outside of prison and 33% of offenders reported that they have attended examinations and routine dental treatments inside prison [11] have permitted the research questions to be raised about the role of Cohen's [16] accessibility factors as explanatory elements for offenders when they access dental services inside prison.

Cohen [16], in her seminal paper on accessing dental services, suggested that accessibility factors relating specifically to the patient include dental anxiety, costs of treatment, and perceived need. These factors could either enable or inhibit a person's access to dental services. Some 30 years later, Marshman et al. [17] revisited the issues of accessibility and showed that, in relation to the patient, the perception of treatment need has remained an important accessibility factor. Focusing on people in prison and their access to prison dental services, Marshman et al. [18] proposed that their perception of dental need, together with their pattern of routine dental attendance outside of prison, has enabled prisoners to engage in routine attendance inside prison. However, the role of perceived need was, according to Marshman et al. [18], found to be poorly associated with accessing prison dental services. Their work [18] seemed to suggest that a person's pattern of dental services' attendance outside of prison had a stronger influence upon accessing dental services in prison than their perception of dental need. The research of Marshman et al. [18] thus supported the hypothesis that there must be additional and intervening accessibility factors, such as prison experience, which could influence the utilization of prison dental services. This hypothesis is timely and appropriate, because accessible health services are considered to be of central importance in the promotion of prisoner health [8–10]. The following research question remains, however: what are these additional and intervening accessibility factors that affect the utilization of prison dental services during custodial sentences? Therefore, the aim of this study was to conduct an oral health and psychosocial needs survey to identify factors associated with accessing prison dental services in Scotland.

2. Methods

2.1. Sample

The 3 Scottish prisons were chosen for participation from the prison estate because, [i] they were representative of a maximum security prison for adult male offenders, a prison for women, and female young offenders and a male young offenders' institution, and [ii] they all had National Health Services dental treatment. The dental treatment provided in the prison setting includes restorative dentistry (conservation and prosthetic and endodontic treatments), the extraction of teeth, preventive dental treatments (e.g., scale and polish), and emergency dental care. The prisoners all had a visiting dentist who provided treatment; however, the availability of such services was affected by security checks, restrictions on movement, finding prison officers to escort prisoners to and from the dental surgery, and competing priorities within the prison environment [19].

A non-probability convenience sample of offenders from these 3 prisons was obtained. A post-hoc power analysis confirmed that a sample size of 250 would give 80% power to detect a one-sided significant increase in the reported prison dental services' attendance of 9% when the reference category reported a baseline attendance of 45% [20].

The ethical committees required that all the prisoners were to have the same opportunity to participate, and thus, a non-probability sampling technique was appropriate. Offenders, nevertheless, who were assessed by prison staff to pose a risk to the researchers and those who did not understand English were excluded from the survey. Informed consent was obtained from all the prisoners taking part in the survey.

2.2. Questionnaire

The questionnaire consisted of the following features.

i. Demographic Profile of the Participants

The first part of the questionnaire gathered information about the participants' demographic profile, including age in years and gender, previous occupation prior to imprisonment, and prison experience, which included the total length of time in prison, amount of time on remand, and number of prison sentences.

ii. Dental Anxiety Status: The Modified Dental Anxiety Scale (MDAS)

Dental anxiety was assessed using the Modified Dental Anxiety Scale (MDAS). MDAS consists of 5 questions. It asks the participants how anxious they feel regarding waiting for dental treatment, drilling, scaling and polishing, and local anesthesia. The respondents rate their dental anxiety on a 5-point scale, which ranges from not anxious (1) to extremely anxious (5). Possible scores range from 5 to 25, with scores over 19 indicating dental phobia. The normative value for the general population in the United Kingdom is 12.0 [21,22]. The MDAS has good reliability with a Cronbach's alpha of 0.93 [23]. The Cronbach's alpha was 0.94 for this sample of people in prison.

iii. Oral Health-Related Quality of Life: The Oral Health Impact Scale-14 (OHIP-14)

The OHIP-14 is a 14-item inventory that assesses oral health-related quality of life. It is based on a hierarchy of impacts arising from oral disease, ranging in severity, and it includes questions on functional limitations (e.g., pronouncing words), physical pain (e.g., painful, aching mouth), psychological discomfort (e.g., feeling self-conscious), physical disability (e.g., interrupted meals), psychological disability (e.g., feeling embarrassed), social disability (e.g., irritable with others), and handicap (e.g., life less satisfying). The respondents were asked how frequently they had experienced each of the oral impacts in the previous 12 months with questions such as 'Have you had painful aching in your mouth'. The responses were made on a 5-point Likert scale, with scores ranging from 0 (never) to 4 (very often) [24]. OHIP-14 has good reliability with a Cronbach's alpha of 0.91 [25]. The Cronbach's alpha for the total OHIP-14 score was 0.95 for this sample of people in prison.

iv. Reported Dental Services' Attendance Behavior

The final part of the questionnaire asked about access to prison dental services during imprisonment, either for an emergency or a dental examination and routine dental treatments [26]. This was a simple dichotomous variable. In addition, the offenders were asked about their usual pattern of dental services' attendance outside of prison.

2.3. Training for the Administration of the Questionnaire and the Oral Health Examination

Prior to the survey, which took place between September and December 2011, the research team, including the two participating dentists and dental nurses, were trained in the adoption of the operational protocols to gain consent and gather data in the prison setting, as well as breakout training. Breakout training ensured that in the event of a disturbance, the research team would be safe. Training by a health psychologist on how to assist the participants, as required, with the completion of the questionnaire without influencing their responses was also provided.

The dental examiners were specifically chosen, because they had recently been calibrated for a national oral health survey with percentage agreements in the range of 91–100% and a Kappa of >0.8 [27]. They were also chosen because they had experience working in the prison sector. The International Caries Detection and Assessment System (ICDAS) is a clinical, visual scoring system for obvious dental decay [28,29]. In the ICDAS nomenclature, decay is described as D_1MFT and includes all white spots, brown spots, enamel, and dentine cavitated lesions (ICDAS caries codes 1, 2, 3, 4, 5, or 6). D_2MFT includes all enamel and dentine cavitated lesions (ICDAS caries codes 3, 4, 5, or 6), and D_3MFT includes only dentinal cavitated lesions (ICDAS caries codes 3, 4, 5, or 6). ICDAS standardization exercises using the ICDAS criteria for detecting caries [29] were provided by Professor Gail Douglas, the ICDAS coordinator. For ICDAS, the percentage difference in the detection of the category obvious decay ($D_{3cv}MFT$ ICDAS caries codes 3–5) between the two dental examiners was 4%, showing a high degree of equivalence ($P = 0.34$). For the purposes of this oral health needs assessment, ICDAS was used to diagnose obvious decay, and the ICDAS findings were converted to $D_{3cv}MFT$, that is, carious lesions that were dentinal, cavitated (c), and visual (v) [30].

2.4. Data Collection Procedure

The participants were asked to complete the questionnaire prior to the dental examination. Assistance was provided to those participants who experienced reading difficulty when completing the survey. This assistance did not influence the participants' responses, as instructed on the training day. The dental examination took place once the questionnaire was completed. The dental examination was conducted in the prison residential areas with infection control procedures observed. A Daray versatile medical light, as in the National Dental Inspection Programmes [26], was used. The 2 dental nurses assisted with the clinical data collection.

2.5. Ethical Issues and Procedures

Ethical approval was obtained from the National Research Ethics Service (reference number NRES 10/S0501/10) and the Scottish Prison Service Ethics Committee. All the data files were held securely on encrypted University computers, and the transcriptions were stored in a secure location. A coding system was used to anonymize the prisoners' data.

2.6. Statistical Analysis

The data were entered into a database and analyzed using SPSS v21 and STAT v13. The data were subjected to frequency distributions, Cronbach's alpha, chi-squared analyses, and t-tests. A hierarchical multivariable logistic regression analysis was undertaken to characterize the offenders who said they had accessed dental services within the prison estate, either for an emergency or routine dental examination and/or treatment appointment during their imprisonment. The 'xtmelogit' procedure was used to enable control of the clustering variable, namely, the prison of confinement. The intra-class correlation coefficient was calculated to determine the level of clustering. The dependent variable was access to dental services when in prison with 'no' coded as 0 and 'yes' coded as 1. The independent variables were age (in years) and number of prison remands, which were entered into the analysis as Model 1. The remaining independent variables were sequentially included in the analysis as follows: OHIP item 'feeling irritable with people because of teeth, mouth, or dentures', pattern of dental attendance outside of prison (emergency = 0: routine = 1), teeth decayed into dentine, and missing teeth.

3. Results

3.1. The Sample

A convenience sample of 342 prisoners (243 males, 99 females) from the three Scottish prisons participated. All the participants completed the questionnaire, and 87% (208 males, 90 females) had an oral examination. A total of 44 prisoners did not take part in the oral health examination for the following reasons: refusal to be examined (25%), attendance at court (25%), discharged/preparing for discharge from prison (11%), at work/education (14%), moved to another prison (9%), and agency visit (5%). There was no significant difference in the proportion of male and female offenders who participated and did not participate in the oral examination ($X^2[1] = 1.11$: $P = 0.18$). All the missing data were excluded, providing a valid response rate of 76% (259). The statistical analysis was conducted on the 259 complete datasets.

3.2. Demographic Profile

The mean age for the participants was 27.21 (± 9.80) years. A total of 29% (76) were female. Additionally, 66% (172) were unemployed and not working prior to imprisonment; of the remainder, 75 were in some form of employment, 8 were in training, and 4 were in full-time education. The majority was Caucasian (94%). Over 80% (211) were single.

3.3. Prison Experience

The total length of time spent in prison while sentenced ranged from 1 day to 34 years, with an average of 2.02 (± 4.14) years. The mean number of remands was 3.84 (± 4.93), and the mean number of prison sentences was 2.63 (± 3.88). The mean length of time spent in prison, during their current sentence at the time of the survey, was 4.93 (± 3.88) months.

3.4. Reported Dental Services' Attendance

A total of 54% (141) of offenders stated that their usual pattern of dental services' attendance outside of prison was for the relief of pain (emergency care). A total of 46% (118) of participants stated that they had attended the prison dentist during their sentences. Of the 118 prisoners who reported that they had accessed prison dental services, 55% said that they had accessed dental services only in an emergency, and 33% stated that they had attended for a dental examination and routine treatment. The reported treatment received during imprisonment, included restorations (93%); extractions (68%); scaling and polishing (66%); teeth crowns (26%), and treatment for dentures (18%). The offenders who had accessed prison dental services were significantly older than those who had not ($t = 4.91$: $P < 0.001$). Prisoners with a significantly greater mean total years of imprisonment ($t = 6.24$: $P < 0.001$) and those with a significantly greater mean number of times in remand ($t = 2.35$: $P = 0.02$) had accessed dental services more often compared with others. For prisoners who had not accessed prisoner dental services, they stated that the barriers to attending prison dental services during imprisonment were difficulty in arranging an appointment (61%), infrequent clinics (48%), and problems getting (10%) and completing (3%) prison request forms.

3.5. Oral Health-Related Attitudes

3.5.1. Dental Anxiety

The mean score for dental anxiety was 10.02 (± 5.56). There were no significant differences in total mean MDAS scores between those participants who had accessed dental services in the prison setting (10.22 $\pm$ 5.59) and those who had not (9.86 $\pm$ 5.54) ($t = 0.52$: $P = 0.60$).

3.5.2. Oral Health-Related Quality of Life

The mean OHIP-14 score was 15.61 (± 14.34) with a range from 0 to 56. There was a significant difference in the total mean OHIP-14 score between those who had accessed dental services in prison (18.37 $\pm$ 14.97) and those who had not (13.20 $\pm$ 13.35) ($t = 2.81$: $P = 0.005$). Table 1 shows the statistically significant differences between the mean scores for the oral health impact items between those who had accessed and those who had not accessed dental services in the prison setting (Table 1). There were no statistically significant differences in mean scores for OHIP items between male, female, and young offenders.

Table 1. Comparison of Oral Health Impact Scale (OHIP) items by access to prison dental services.

Oral Health-Related Quality of Life	Accessed Prison Dental Services		t	P
OHIP Item	Yes (n = 118) x (SD)	No (n = 141) x (SD)		
uncomfortable eating	1.26 (1.33)	1.69 (1.50)	2.40	0.02
self-conscious about appearance	1.47 (1.52)	2.09 (1.59)	3.20	0.002
feeling tense about appearance	1.31 (1.40)	1.76 (1.53)	2.34	0.02
unsatisfactory diet	0.60 (1.00)	0.99 (1.34)	2.60	0.01
interrupted meals	0.76 (1.17)	1.26 (1.38)	3.27	0.001
difficulty relaxing	1.05 (1.29)	1.48 (1.42)	2.50	0.01
embarrassed about appearance	1.44 (1.57)	1.94 (1.66)	2.46	0.01
irritable with others	0.83 (1.25)	1.34 (1.45)	2.98	0.003
difficulty doing usual jobs	0.51 (0.96)	0.88 (1.26)	2.47	0.01
feeling unable to function	0.54 (1.03)	0.85 (1.26)	2.11	0.04

3.6. Obvious Decay Experience

Only 10 participants had no obvious signs of dental caries experience. The remainder of the sample had experience of dental caries. For the entire sample (n = 259), the mean number of decayed, missing, and filled teeth ($D_{3cv}MFT$) was 10.21 (± 6.32); the mean number of decayed teeth (D_{3cv}) was 1.62 (SD $\pm$ 2.22); the mean number of missing teeth was 4.36 (± 4.45); and the mean number of filled teeth was 4.23 (± 3.80). The participants who had accessed dental services in the prison setting had a significantly greater mean $D_{3cv}MFT$, a significantly greater mean number of missing teeth, and a significantly greater mean number of filled teeth (Table 2). More offenders (62%) who had not accessed prison dental services had teeth decayed into dentine than those who had accessed dental services in the prison setting (38%) ($X^2[1] = 5.64$: P = 0.02), and the difference was statistically significant.

Table 2. Mean score of $D_{3cv}MFT$, decayed, missing, and filled teeth in this Scottish prisoner population.

Accessed Dental Services in Prison	Decayed Teeth Mean (SD)	Missing Teeth Mean (SD)	Filled Teeth Mean (SD)	$D_{3cv}MFT$ Mean (SD)
Yes (n = 118)	1.36 (2.10)	5.93 (4.91)	4.93 (3.69)	12.22 (6.39)
No (n = 141)	1.84 (2.30)	3.05 (3.55)	3.65 (3.80)	8.54 (5.76)
t	1.78	5.32	2.75	4.82
P	0.08	<0.001	0.006	<0.001

3.7. Identifying Factors Associated with Access to Prison Dental Services

Table 3 shows the hierarchical multivariable logistic regression analysis, which was conducted to identify factors associated with access to prison dental services. A Poisson regression with a robust variance estimator was also performed, and the results were inspected. No appreciable differences in the substantial effects were found. Hence, the logistic model was selected for ease of presentation. An analysis was conducted to compute the intra-class correlation, which was found to be 0.114: [95 %CI: 0.021, 0.438]: $X^2[1] = 19.33$, P < 0.001. Hence, all the regression results presented have been controlled for clustering due to prison membership, preventing biased parameter estimates. It was decided, in addition, to omit gender in the regression, as this was already implicated within the prison category. Age and prison experience were entered into the analysis as Step 1. Model 1 characterized the offenders by demography and prison experience (remand) and explained 19% of the variance. Model 2, while controlling for demography and prison experience, showed that an offender was 36% more likely to attend dental services for every unit change in the 5-point ranking scale of 'feeling irritable with people because of teeth, mouth, or dentures' and explained an additional 7% of the variance. Model 3 was adopted as the final model to characterize offenders who accessed dental services when in prison and explained an additional 9% of the variance. Model 3 therefore explained a total of 35% of the variance. Consequently, an offender who accessed dental care during his/her imprisonment had an 8% increased likelihood of attending for every experience of remand, a 32% increased likelihood of accessing dental services for each increased level of irritability, and an over 2 times greater chance of emergency dental services' attendance. Furthermore, there was an 18% lower chance of accessing dental services for each additional tooth affected by decay, and a 13% greater likelihood of accessing dental services for each unit increase in missing teeth.

Table 3. Identifying factors associated with access to prison dental services.

Factors Associated with Accessing Services	Model 1			Model 2			Model 3		
	OR	95 %CI	P	OR	95% CI	P	OR	95% CI	P
Age (in years)	1.05	1.01, 1.09	0.006	1.05	1.02, 1.09	<0.004	1.03	0.99, 1.07	0.20
Prison experience (number of times in remand)	1.06	1.00, 1.14	0.04	1.05	0.99, 1.12	0.004	1.08	1.01, 1.16	0.03
OHIP: irritable with people				1.36	1.11, 1.66	0.003	1.32	1.06, 1.66	0.02
Pattern of dental attendance outside of prison: routine							1		
emergency							2.17	1.19, 3.93	0.01
Total number of decayed teeth (D3_{cv}T)							0.82	0.70, 0.95	0.01
Total number of missing teeth (MT)							1.13	1.04, 1.22	0.004
Variance explained	19%			26%			35%		
−2 log likelihood	164.89			151.97			147.68		
df	3			4			7		
ΔX² (Δdf)				9.30 (1)			20.58 (3)		
P				0.002			<0.001		

Model 1: Adjusted for age and prison remands. Model 2: Adjusted for variables in Model 1 plus OHIP item 'feeling irritable with people because of teeth, mouth, or dentures'. Model 3: Adjusted for variable in Model 2 plus pattern of dental attendance outside of prison, total number of D3_{cv}T, and total number of MT.

4. Discussion

The aim of this work was to conduct an oral health and psychosocial needs survey to identify factors associated with accessing prison dental service. The results of the survey identified accessibility factors that characterized the utilization of prison dental services during custodial sentences.

The access of people in custody to prison dental services was the main concern of this study. Because the definition of dental services' utilization is a combination of associated accessibility factors, it is of importance to identify them and to illustrate how different reasons for accessing dental services may be informative. This study demonstrated that for people in custody, the associated accessibility factors when utilizing dental services were in some ways different to those in the general population [16–18]

The predominant accessibility or associated factors that influenced the utilization of prison dental services were age and prison experience (i.e., the number of times in remand). While it is to be expected that longer time in prison would be associated with increased reported access to prison dental services, the mean length of the participating offenders' current sentences was merely 4.93 months, which was equivalent to the national average sentence length of 4 months [23]. Because attendance could be argued to be a prevalence variable, it may be suggested that an individual whose custodial sentence was 8 months (rather than the 4-month average) would have had twice as much opportunity to access dental care; however, we contend that the above observation indicated that another prison experience factor, in addition to the length of time of the current imprisonment, influenced access to prison dental services. We postulate that because the literature suggests that poor health literacy affects access to health services [12–15], then an alternative means of gaining information on how to access services must exist. We speculate that increased experience of prison remand could have provided an environment in which the offenders gained information on and knowledge of how to access dental services—whether this was for emergency or routine care [11]. Although oral health-related quality of life differentiated between those who had and had not accessed prison dental services, the same was not so for dental anxiety. Moreover, the mean number of teeth decayed into dentine was 1.62 teeth; however, only 46% had accessed prison dental services—suggesting that this unmet treatment need, as proposed by Marshman et al. [18], had not acted to prompt the offenders to access dental care. Considering that oral health impacts differentiated between those who had and had not accessed prison dental services, we again speculate that when prisoners' oral health impacts their quality of life, then offenders access prison dental services.

We suggest that the results of the hierarchical multivariable logistic regression analysis support our proposition that an intervening oral health-related quality of life variable increased the offenders' awareness of their dental needs and enabled access to dental treatment. We propose this because the findings showed that greater experience of prison remand and the impact of oral health upon irritability with others, together with a greater mean number of missing teeth but a lower mean number of decayed teeth, characterized those who accessed prison dental services. The proposition that an association exists between oral health and its impact upon quality of life, which, in turn, raises awareness of perceived need and thus improves access to dental services, is also supported by the work of others [7,14,18]. It is interesting that this specific oral impact—increased irritability with others—appeared to act as a trigger to increase the utilization of prison dental services. This suggestion finds support in the finding that those who had accessed dental services had lower mean scores for irritability. This is the first time that an investigation has shown that the oral health impact of irritability with others (social disability) outweighed dental indifference in a prison population, as reflected in this OHIP item's ability to increase the explanation of the model. Although this work was conducted in Scottish prisons with a non-probability convenience sample, the finding that the prisoners were irritable with others on account of their teeth is worrisome and should be of interest to anyone working in the prison environment [1–3,7,17,18,28].

There are limitations to this work. First, the sample is a non-probability convenience sample, and consequently, there are implications regarding the representativeness of the sample. The mean length of sentence for this sample of prisoners was 4.93 months, which is equivalent to the 4-month Scottish average for a custodial sentence (23); therefore, it may be suggested that, with regard to the average length of sentence, they were equivalent to other prison populations and national averages. In this convenience sample of prisoners, 46% reported they had accessed prison dental services, which approximates to the 43% found by Marshman et al. [18] and the 50% found by Rodrigues et al. [7]. Secondly, this is a cross-sectional survey, and the limitations surrounding the use of such data is acknowledged here, together with the need for additional work to confirm the findings presented here. Therefore, with regard to the reported access to care, this sample was commensurate with others in the United Kingdom and South America. Thirdly, although the dental examiners had been calibrated for a recent national dental survey, they were standardized for ICDAS. This was a potential source of error. However, there was a high degree of equivalence in the detection of obvious decay between the examiners, suggesting that the oral health findings were trustworthy. Finally, the OHIP scores were not known before the people in custody had or had not accessed prison dental services and is, therefore, a potential limitation. Thus, although the findings of this work must be interpreted with caution, they nonetheless highlight the importance of accessibility factors and, in particular, health literacy and irritability with others as additional and intervening factors in reported access to prison dental services.

This survey identified and characterized access to prison dental services during custodial sentences. Of particular interest is the proposition that when oral health impacts quality of life, there appears to be increased awareness of the need for dental health treatment, which, in turn, promotes dental services' attendance. These findings should be of interest to all those who work within the prison sector [31]. Allen et al. [32] have proposed the need to have 'cross-sector collaborations' when providing health care to reduce health inequity. This type of cross-sector collaboration is now in existence in Scotland in the form of the oral health promotion intervention for people in custody through a program called 'Mouth Matters'. Mouth Matters represents a cross-sector collaboration between the Scottish Health Boards and the Scottish Prison Service [33]. This investigation provides additional support for 'cross-sector collaboration' and the need to work in partnership with those from the prison services, health-care colleagues, and those in custody to improve the oral health, health literacy, and the oral health-related quality of life of people in prison.

5. Conclusions

In conclusion, this investigation identified factors associated with access to prison dental services in Scotland. The role of accessibility factors, such as the oral health impact of irritability, appeared to increase perceptions of dental need and promote the attendance of dental services.

Author Contributions: R.F. and D.R. were the principal investigators of the survey. R.F. and D.R. conceptualized and wrote the manuscript. R.F. and D.R. revised the manuscript.

Funding: The authors are thankful for funding from the Scottish Government (award number: 121.804485).

Conflicts of Interest: The authors declare no conflict of interest.

References

1. Heidari, E.; Dickson, C.; Newton, T. An overview of the prison population and the general health status of prisoners. *Br. Dent. J.* **2014**, *217*, 15–19. [CrossRef] [PubMed]
2. Akaji, E.; Ashiwaju, M. Oral health status of a sample of prisoners in Enugu: A disadvantaged population. *Ann. Med. Health Sci. Res.* **2014**, *4*, 650–653. [CrossRef] [PubMed]
3. Osborn, M.; Butler, T.; Barnard, P.D. Oral health status of prison inmates—New South Wales, Australia. *Aust. Dent. J.* **2003**, *48*, 34–38. [CrossRef] [PubMed]
4. Guarnizo-Herreño, C.C.; Watt, R.G.; Fuller, E.; Steele, J.G.; Shen, J.; Morris, S.; Wildman, J.; Tsakos, G. Socioeconomic position and subjective oral health: Findings for the adult population in England, Wales and Northern Ireland. *BMC Public Health* **2014**, *14*, 827. [CrossRef] [PubMed]

5. Jones, C.; McCann, M.; Nugent, Z. Scottish Prisons Dental Health Survey 2002. Available online: http://www.scotland.gov.uk/Resource/Doc/47210/0013527.pdf (accessed on 6 February 2004).
6. Heidari, E.; Dickinson, C.; Wilson, R.; Fiske, J. Oral health of remand prisoners in HMP Brixton, London. *Br. Dent. J.* **2007**, *202*. [CrossRef] [PubMed]
7. Rodrigues, I.S.; Silveira, I.T.; Pinto, M.S.; Xavier, A.F.; de Oliveira, T.B.; de Paiva, S.M.; de Castro, R.D.; Cavalcanti, A.L. Locked mouths: Tooth loss in a women's prison in northeastern Brazil. *Sci. World J.* **2014**, *2014*. [CrossRef] [PubMed]
8. World Health Organization. Europe Guide on Prison and Health. Available online: http://www.euro.who.int/en/health-topics/health-determinants/prisons-andhealth/publications/2014/prisons-and-health (accessed on 24 May 2010).
9. Brutus, L.; Mackie, P.; Millard, A.; Fraser, A.; Conacher, A.; Hardie, S.; McDowall, L.; Meechan, H. Better Health, Better Lives for Prisoners: A Framework for Improving the Health of Scotland's Prisoners: Volume 1: The Framework. ScotPHN, Glasgow, 2012. Available online: http://www.scotphn.net/pdf/2012_06_08_Health_improvement_for_prisoners_vol_1_Final_(Web_version)1.pdf (accessed on 15 January 2013).
10. Everington, T. Healthier People Safer Communities: Working Together to Improve Outcomes for Offenders. Available online: https://www.scotphn.net/wp-content/uploads/2015/10/Healthier-People-Safer-Communities-April-2013.pdf (accessed on 2 September 2013).
11. Freeman, R.; Akbar, T.; Buls, D.; Edwards, M.; Everington, T.; Richards, D.; Themessl-Huber, M.; Watt, C. The Oral Health and Psychosocial Needs of Scottish Prisoners and Young Offenders. Available online: http://dentistry.dundee.ac.uk/sites/dentistry.dundee.ac.uk/files/media/SOHIPP-report.pdf (accessed on 25 September 2012).
12. Donelle, L.; Hall, J. An exploration of women offenders' health literacy. *Soc. Work Public Health* **2014**, *29*, 240–251. [CrossRef] [PubMed]
13. Heidari, E.; Dickinson, C.; Newton, T. Multidisciplinary team working in an adult male prison establishment in the UK. *Br. Dent. J.* **2014**, *217*, 117–121. [CrossRef] [PubMed]
14. Buunk-Werkhoven, Y.A.; Dijkstra, A.; Schaub, R.M.; van der Schans, C.P.; Spreen, M. Oral health related quality of life among imprisoned Dutch forensic psychiatric patients. *J. Forensic. Nurs.* **2010**, *6*, 137–143. [CrossRef] [PubMed]
15. Vacca, J.S. Educated prisoners are less likely to return to prison. *J. Correct. Educ.* **2004**, *55*, 297–305.
16. Cohen, L.K. Converting unmet need for care to effective demand. *Int. Dent. J.* **1987**, *37*, 114–116. [PubMed]
17. Marshman, Z.; Porritt, J.; Dyer, T.; Wyborn, C.; Godson, J.; Baker, S. What influences the use of dental services by adults in the UK? *Community Dent. Oral Epidemiol.* **2012**, *40*, 306–314. [CrossRef] [PubMed]
18. Marshman, Z.; Baker, S.R.; Robinson, P.G. Does dental indifference influence the oral health-related quality of life of prisoners? *Community Dent. Oral Epidemiol.* **2014**, *42*, 470–480. [CrossRef] [PubMed]
19. Smith, P.A.; Themessl-Huber, M.; Akbar, T.; Richards, D.; Freeman, R. What motivates dentists to work in prisons? A qualitative exploration. *Br. Dent. J.* **2011**, *211*, E7. [CrossRef] [PubMed]
20. Gillett, R. Post hoc power analysis. *J. Appl. Psychol.* **1994**, *79*, 783–785. [CrossRef]
21. Hill, K.B.; Chadwick, B.; Freeman, R.; O'Sullivan, I.; Murray, J.J. Adult Dental Health Survey 2009: Relationships between dental attendance patterns, oral health behaviour and the current barriers to dental care. *Br. Dent. J.* **2013**, *214*. [CrossRef] [PubMed]
22. Humphris, G.M.; Crawford, J.R.; Hill, K.; Gilbert, A.; Freeman, R. UK Population Norms for the Modified Dental Anxiety Scale with Percentile Calculator: Adult Dental Health Survey 2009 Results. *BMC Oral Health* **2013**, *13*. [CrossRef] [PubMed]
23. Newton, J.T.; Edwards, J.C. Psychometric properties of the modified dental anxiety scale: An independent replication. *Community Dent. Health* **2005**, *22*, 40–42. [PubMed]
24. Locker, D.; Allen, P.F. Developing short-form measures of oral health-related quality of life. *J. Public Health Dent.* **2002**, *62*, 13–20. [CrossRef] [PubMed]
25. Robinson, P.G.; Gibson, B.; Khan, F.A.; Birnbaum, W. Validity of two oral health-related quality of life measures. *Community Dent. Oral Epidemiol.* **2003**, *31*, 90–99. [CrossRef] [PubMed]
26. Scottish Government. Prison Statistics and Population Projections Scotland: 2011-12. Available online: http://www.scotland.gov.uk/Resource/0039/00396363.pdf (accessed on 29 June 2012).

27. NHS National Services Scotland. National Dental Inspection Programme. Available online: http://www.isdscotland.org/Health-Topics/Dental-Care/National-Dental-Inspection-Programme/ (accessed on 29 October 2018).
28. Ismail, A.I.; Sohn, W.; Tellez, M.; Amaya, A.; Sen, A.; Hasson, H.; Pitts, N.B. The International Caries Detection and Assessment System (ICDAS): An Integrated System for Measuring Dental Caries. *Community Dent. Oral Epidemiol.* **2007**, *35*, 170–178. [CrossRef] [PubMed]
29. ICDAS Foundation. International Caries Detection and Assessment System. Available online: https://www.icdas.org/ (accessed on 25 September 2012).
30. International Caries Detection and Assessment System (ICDAS) Coordinating Committee. Criteria Manual International Caries Detection and Assessment System. Available online: https://www.icdas.org/uploads/ICDAS%20Criteria%20Document%20corrected%202013.pdf (accessed on 25 September 2012).
31. Costa, J. Dental care in corrections. *Dis. Mon.* **2014**, *60*, 221–223. [CrossRef] [PubMed]
32. Allen, J.; Goldblatt, P.; Daly, S.; Jabbal, J.; Marmot, M. Reducing Health Inequalities through New Models of Care: A Resource for New Care Models. 2018. Available online: http://www.instituteofhealthequity.org/resources-reports/reducing-health-inequalities-through-new-models-of-care-a-resource-for-new-care-models (accessed on 8 January 2019).
33. NHS Health Scotland. Mouth Matters Guide to Trainers: Better Oral Care for Offenders. Available online: http://www.knowledge.scot.nhs.uk/media/CLT/ResourceUploads/4086716/a2b802de-6f65-4594-b749-01cfe0f5b9e4.pdf (accessed on 10 December 2018).

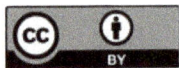

© 2019 by the authors. Licensee MDPI, Basel, Switzerland. This article is an open access article distributed under the terms and conditions of the Creative Commons Attribution (CC BY) license (http://creativecommons.org/licenses/by/4.0/).

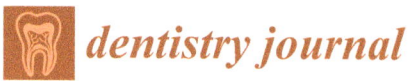

Article

Implementing an Oral Health Intervention for People Experiencing Homelessness in Scotland: A Participant Observation Study

Laura Beaton [1,*], Isobel Anderson [2], Gerry Humphris [3], Andrea Rodriguez [1] and Ruth Freeman [1]

1. Dental Health Services Research Unit, School of Dentistry, University of Dundee, Dundee DD1 4HN, Scotland, UK; a.rodriguez@dundee.ac.uk (A.R.); R.E.Freeman@dundee.ac.uk (R.F.)
2. Housing Studies, Faculty of Social Sciences, University of Stirling, Stirling FK9 4LA, Scotland, UK; isobel.anderson@stir.ac.uk
3. School of Medicine, Medical & Biological Sciences, University of St Andrews, North Haugh, St Andrews KY16 9TF, Scotland, UK; gmh4@st-andrews.ac.uk
* Correspondence: l.z.beaton@dundee.ac.uk Tel: +44-(0)-138-274-0917

Received: 3 October 2018; Accepted: 19 November 2018; Published: 1 December 2018

Abstract: Smile4life is an intervention aimed at improving the oral health of people experiencing homelessness in Scotland. The purpose of this research was to determine how this intervention was being translated from guidance into action. Data concerning Smile4life working practices were collected in three NHS Boards using participant observation. Fieldnotes taken during these observations were analysed using content analysis. This analysis revealed that there were working alliances between the oral health practitioner, the Third Sector staff, and the homeless service users, and that these alliances were affected by various barriers and enablers. The observation sessions also highlighted variations in working practices.

Keywords: homeless persons; oral health; delivery of health care; dental health services

1. Introduction

Homelessness is a multi-dimensional experience characterised not merely by the lack of a roof over one's head but also by physiological and emotional deprivation [1]. Being homeless can be "impoverishing and isolating" and is often associated with physical and mental ill-health [2]. Indeed, as Scottish Government statistics show, 42% of those who were assessed as homeless during 2015–2016 were found to have one or more additional support needs, including mental ill-health, drug or alcohol dependency as well as medical condition(s) [3]. This suggests that this group of people had experienced multiple exclusion homelessness, which can be defined as the experience of homelessness in addition to one or more of the following: institutional care (e.g., prison, hospital or being a looked after child); street activities such as begging; or substance misuse [4].

In addition to the physical health of people experiencing homelessness, there is evidence that this population have poor oral health. Previous studies have found that homeless populations have a high prevalence of bleeding gums, calculus and periodontal inflammation [5–7]. Research has also found that people experiencing homelessness often have a poor record of dental attendance and unmet treatment needs [6]. In addition, this population has been found to suffer from dental anxiety and poor oral health related quality of life [5].

People experiencing homelessness face many health inequalities—for example, they have a higher risk of death than the general population, as well as higher rates of suicide and depression [8]. Poor oral health could also be seen as a contributing factor to the health inequalities faced by the homeless population: the Groundswell Healthy Mouths report found that "participants were regularly facing issues with their oral health that were making it difficult for them to live fulfilled lives" [9] (p. 2). In addition, those that had oral health problems reported being "handicapped" with 21% of participants reporting they felt "completely unable to function" because of their oral health, compared to 1% of the general population [9] (p. 2). Many reported turning to alcohol and drugs to help them cope with their dental pain, which, in turn, exacerbates other health needs [8].

The Scottish Government recognised the health needs of the Scottish homeless population in 2005, with the Health and Homelessness Standards, designed to improve the health of people experiencing homelessness and to tackle health inequalities [10]. This was followed in the same year by the Dental Action Plan, which recognised people experiencing homelessness as a priority group that required tailored oral healthcare [11]. Both documents called for the National Health Service (NHS) to take steps to address the general and oral health of people experiencing homelessness in Scotland. In Scotland, the NHS is comprised of 14 Boards, each linked to a geographical area of the country, and provides primary and secondary healthcare to the whole population, regardless of their ability to pay, and is free at the point of delivery [12]. This need for tailored health messages was strengthened by evidence from a systematic review and meta-analysis that concluded that messages that were tailored to the health needs of patients were effective in promoting behaviour change [13]. In 2012, the Scottish Government renewed its commitment to the oral health of people experiencing homelessness in the Priority Groups Strategy, which emphasised the need for accessible dental services and preventive oral health programmes [14].

In response to the Scottish Government's policies, an oral health intervention, called Smile4life, was developed to address the oral health needs of the homeless population in Scotland. It was developed from the evidence-base gleaned from a national survey of 853 participants that was conducted during 2008–2009. This sample population was shown to have had poorer oral and psychosocial health when compared to the general population of Scotland [15]. Qualitative interviews also took place with 34 people experiencing homelessness, highlighting that maintaining good oral health was not always practically possible when homeless. Furthermore, oral health was often not a priority, as evidenced by poor dental attendance [15]. Together, the quantitative and qualitative findings from the Smile4life report led to the development of the Smile4life intervention and accompanying Guide for Trainers [16], a resource intended to be used by National Health Service (NHS) and Third Sector staff to assist in the training of their staff to deliver evidence-based oral health messages to their service users. For the purposes of this research, the Third Sector refers to voluntary or charity organisations or community groups working with homeless service users, providing support and/or accommodation.

The Guide for Trainers provided oral health practitioners and Third Sector staff with: an overview of homelessness and oral health, including barriers and enablers to oral health care; information about oral health (e.g., specific problems, access to care, and preventive care advice); information about the common risk factor approach to oral health; and information about the Smile4life intervention itself, including guidelines for specific roles that practitioners could adopt, motivational interviewing techniques, how to deliver tailored oral health advice, and how to support behaviour change. The Guide for Trainers, and the Smile4life intervention itself, was launched in 2012 [16].

A theory-based process evaluation of the implementation of the Smile4life intervention began in 2013. Regular telephone interviews took place with NHS staff responsible for the implementation. The evaluation found that it took NHS Boards an average of 16 months to implement the Smile4life intervention following the launch of the Guide for Trainers training package. The results of this evaluation highlighted various barriers to successful implementation, particularly a lack of resources (staffing, time constraints), and poor engagement between the NHS and the Third Sector [17]. Factors that facilitated implementation included motivated practitioners and a willingness to engage with other organisations [17].

While this process evaluation illustrated factors that act as barriers and/or facilitators to successful implementation, much remained unknown about how and why NHS and Third Sector organisations implement Smile4life. Therefore, this study aimed to answer the question: how is Smile4life being translated from national guidance into practice?

To begin to answer this question, it was crucial to ascertain how the Smile4life intervention was currently being delivered within NHS Boards. In order to do so, it was necessary to observe the behaviours associated with the delivery of Smile4life.

2. Materials and Methods

2.1. Sample and Recruitment

Sampling was purposive, with all three NHS Boards being selected because they had taken part in the earlier previous evaluation of Smile4life and had demonstrated contrasting levels of experience and a variety of approaches in delivering oral/dental health services to people affected by homelessness, allowing for a theoretical sampling [17–19]. Furthermore, the NHS Boards also varied in the number of people assessed as being homeless, with Board 3 having 7685, Board 2 having 6056 and Board 1 having 2379 in the most recent statistics from the Scottish Government [20].

The recruited individuals were all NHS employees who worked directly with service users, offered training to Third Sector staff, and delivered oral health education. Their job titles varied depending on the NHS Board of employment and included oral health educators and dental health support workers. Oral health educators promote and raise awareness of oral health issues amongst the homeless population and any Third Sector staff that work in the homelessness sector. They deliver oral health advice, provide support and maintain links with homeless organisations. The role of a dental health support worker is community-based, supporting homeless individuals directly by providing oral health advice, signposting to relevant services, making dental appointments and accompanying patients to the dentist, if required. For the purposes of this article, these participants are referred to as "oral health practitioners".

2.2. Ethical Considerations

Ethical approval was applied for and granted by the University Research Ethics Council at the University of Dundee (UREC 15098). Consent forms had to be read and signed before any observation could take place and all data were anonymised.

2.3. Data Collection

Participant observation was chosen as the data collection method for this research, in order to reveal the existing relationships between the oral health practitioners and Third Sector practitioners and the homeless service users they interact with, as well as variations in the working practices of the oral health practitioners. Participant observation would allow the researcher to observe first hand these interactions and variations as they happened, rather than relying on second-hand accounts from the oral health practitioners themselves about their working practices. Furthermore, using participant observation for this research was in line with Taylor-Powell and Steele's guidelines on when participant observation is appropriate, e.g., "when you are trying to understand ongoing behaviour, process, unfolding situation or event" or "when written or other data collection procedures seem inappropriate" [21] (p. 1). In addition, participant observation is recognised as being a "valuable approach for community health research", providing an opportunity for researchers to become more involved in the community of the person(s) being observed, whereby "the informants are more likely to disclose their real beliefs and perspectives" [22] (p. 4).

Detailed field notes were taken to record what was heard and what was seen. The field notes recorded the date, time and location, as well as any other relevant contextual information, and were written in a narrative style. Notes were made of everything that seemed relevant as Taylor-Powell and

Steele noted "in some situations, observing what does not happen may be as important as observing what happens" [21] (p. 3). Each additional observation session was then informed by the ones that preceded it, allowing for theoretical sampling.

As Jorgensen stated, "it is important at the outset of inquiry to remain open to the unexpected" [23] (p. 82). Therefore, the observation was based on a combination of structured and unstructured formats—there were pre-identified items that should be looked for, as well as space to report anything relevant but unexpected [21]. This allowed an insight into the existing relationship between the oral health practitioners, Third Sector practitioners and homeless service users, and reveal variations in the working practices of the oral health practitioners. It also revealed whether practitioners were following the national guidance in Smile4life, concerning oral health and homelessness.

2.4. Data Analysis

Content analysis was chosen as the method by which to analyse the data collected from the observation sessions. This is a form of data analysis that is understood to be a "systematic and objective means of describing and quantifying phenomena" [24] (p. 108). It "involves establishing categories, (and) systematic linkages between them" [25] (p. 467).

Before any data were collected, the researcher reflected on the aim of the observation sessions—to explore how Smile4life was being delivered within the NHS Boards—and had identified several key topics that would be specifically looked for. The researcher also considered the recommendations made by Mays and Pope that observers should aim "to record exactly what happened, including his or her own feelings and responses to the situations witnessed" [18] (p. 184). The key issues the researcher aimed to observe primarily concerned dialogues about oral health, and the role and skills of the practitioner. The researcher also noted the physical context, any general observations that did not fit into any of these questions, and then her own reflections of the session that had been observed.

These questions helped to select specific areas to examine and analyse, as part of the preparation stage of content analysis, e.g., how practitioners engaged with service users and Third Sector staff, and how they have chosen to implement Smile4life. The data were then open coded—reading through all the field notes and identifying recurrent categories, based on existing knowledge and reflecting on the research question. Memos, written in the margins, were used to note emerging ideas and reflections concerning the data [26]. The process was then repeated, to test and refine and revise categories, with similar sub-categories being grouped together where appropriate [18,27].

3. Results

Data were collected over a ten-month period, beginning in November 2015, and ending in August 2016. Three observation sessions were conducted in Board 1, two in Board 3 and four in Board 2. In Boards 2 and 3, these were whole day sessions, where the researcher accompanied the oral health practitioners to a series of different locations as they went about a normal Smile4life working day. In Board 1, this approach was not possible, so sessions lasted approximately 1.5–2 h—the time that a mobile dental unit spent at a location treating patients. Data were collected at the three locations over a series of sessions until saturation had been reached, i.e., when the researcher had witnessed the full range of services offered by the oral health practitioner being observed. More information about each location visited is provided in Table 1. More details about the practitioners are included in Table 2.

From the initial coding, one overarching theme emerged: a working alliance between the oral health practitioner and (i) the Third Sector staff, and (ii) the service users. Evidence of this alliance is presented below, followed by an exploration of the barriers and enablers to a positive working alliance.

Table 1. Details of observation sessions.

Observation	Location	Services Visited	Setting
Observation 1	Board 2	3 supported accommodation establishments (1 h each)	Shared living room Meeting room
Observation 2	Board 2	An accommodation for young men (1 h) A long-term accommodation for families and individuals (1 h) A short-term accommodation for young people (1 h)	Kitchen Meeting room Shared living room
Observation 3	Board 1	Mobile dental unit at a drop-in service (2 h)	Mobile dental unit waiting area
Observation 4	Board 1	Mobile dental unit at a harm reduction service for young people (1 h 30 min)	Mobile dental unit waiting area
Observation 5	Board 1	Mobile dental unit at a harm reduction service for young people (1 h 30 min)	Mobile dental unit waiting area
Observation 6	Board 2	Drop-in service providing hot meals (3 h)	Canteen
Observation 7	Board 2	A space for families and friend of prisoners to wait before entering the prison (4 h 30 min)	Visitor centre
Observation 8	Board 3	An emergency accommodation for women (1 h) A support and drop-in service (1 h 45 min) An emergency accommodation for men (2 h)	Canteen Reception area
Observation 9	Board 3	A homeless assessment centre and short-term accommodation (2 h) Supported long-term accommodation for women (1 h)	Medical room Service user's flat

Table 2. Details of participating oral health practitioners.

Practitioner Number	Board	Job Title	Gender
Practitioner 3	Board 1	Dental Health Support Worker	Female
Practitioner 1	Board 2	Oral Health Educator	Female
Practitioner 2	Board 2	Oral Health Educator	Female
Practitioner 4	Board 3	Dental Health Support Worker	Female

The concept of a working alliance originated in psychoanalysis, where it is understood to be part of a therapeutic relationship between a health professional and patient. More generally, it is the relationship between a person who wants to make a change, and another person who can help them to make that change [28]. Bordin stated that this working relationship was "key to the change process" [28] (p. 252), and compared the relationship to that of a parent and child or teacher and pupil. Bordin explained that the working alliance is comprised of three factors: "an agreement on goals, an assignment of task or series of tasks, and the development of bonds" [28] (p. 253). In relation to Smile4life, these three factors could be interpreted as: improving the oral health of homeless service users; promoting Smile4life and encouraging service users to attend oral health sessions; and a strong relationship between the oral health practitioner and the Third Sector staff.

It became clear that, with regard to the delivery of Smile4life, the working alliance went beyond the traditional dyadic relationship of a health professional and a patient—it also involved a third element: the Third Sector staff. Triadic relationships first came to prominence in the work of the sociologist Georg Simmel. While Simmel had written about this in 1908, Hill and McGrath [29] argued that it did not gain wider attention until 1950 when his work was definitively translated by Wolf. Simmel stated that when three elements are present "each one operates as an intermediary between the other two" [30] (p. 135). The third person can have three potential roles: (1) a mediator who "deprives conflicting claims of their affective qualities because it neutrally formulates and presents these claims to the two parties involved"; (2) a non-partisan: one party who facilitates the "concord of two colliding parties" or an arbiter who "balances ... contradictory claims against one another"; or (3) a "tertius gaudens", a person that can benefit from the conflict of the other two parties within a triad [30] (pp. 146–154). Simmel also highlighted that, in some situations, a third person joining an existing dyad could be seen as an intruder [30]. Indeed, when two parties are present, there can be no majority but, when a third party joins, the group dynamic can shift to two against one, "revealing emergent power relations" [29] (p. 53).

Within the Smile4life triadic working alliance, there are three principle relationships: (1) the oral health practitioner and the service user; (2) the oral health practitioner and the Third Sector member of staff; and (3) the Third Sector member of staff and the service user. These are discussed in turn below, and are illustrated in Figure 1.

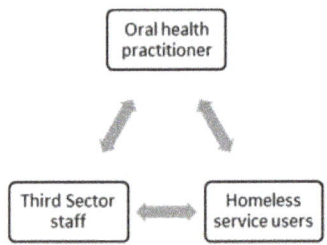

Figure 1. The Smile4life triadic working alliance.

3.1. Alliance 1: Oral Health Practitioner and Service User

For the oral health practitioners that were observed, interacting directly with homeless service users was their main role with regards to delivering the Smile4life intervention (as opposed to training Third Sector staff). Therefore, this alliance needed to be strong, in order for the oral health practitioner to engage with the service users and address their oral health needs, and for the service user to be interested and receptive to the oral health information being discussed. However, this alliance was affected by numerous barriers, which are discussed below.

3.1.1. Barriers

In many of the locations where the oral health practitioners were observed, it was often the oral health practitioner that had the initiative to approach the service user about their oral health, and this was often opportunistic, with the oral health practitioners seizing upon any opportunity to engage with service users.

> *"Practitioner 4 would go up to tables with men having breakfast and say who she was and why she was there, but just to make them aware—it was up to the individuals to approach her if they wanted to"*
>
> *(Observation 8)*

However, as this excerpt from the field notes highlights, the oral health practitioners are dependent on the service users taking an interest in what they have to say. Often, this is not the case—there was occasionally disinterest or hostility from the service users, who were usually not interested in receiving oral health advice. In Boards 2 and 3, many of the interactions with service users are opportunistic, with the oral health practitioner approaching the service user to talk about oral health, rather than the other way around. In one instance, a service user at a drop-in did not want the toothbrush pack from the practitioner because the toothpaste contained fluoride which he considered to be a "neurotoxin". The practitioner tactfully explained the benefits of fluoride, but did not stress the point because the service user was getting angry and argumentative with her.

An additional barrier that prevented the formation of strong working alliance between the oral health practitioners and the service users was the space the oral health practitioner was given by the service in which to deliver Smile4life. As Table 1 shows, in many locations, the oral health practitioner was told to set up in a large communal area, often a canteen—a space in which there is the potential to reach many service users. However, in seven of the services visited, the oral health practitioner was put in a space that meant the service users must approach them, i.e., a medical room, or a meeting room away from the communal spaces. This blocked engagement attempts of any kind, by preventing the oral health practitioner from approaching the service users directly. Furthermore, the rooms the oral health practitioners were put in were predominantly chosen by the staff, and were not always appropriate for the delivery of Smile4life.

> "We were put in the medical room along the corridor from the office, but there was no opportunity for Practitioner 4 to approach any of the residents. We only saw service users if they specifically wanted to talk about their oral health or if they had walked past the room and wanted to see who we were."
>
> (Observation 9)

In the case of Board 1, the space that the oral health practitioners were in was also not ideal, but this was not due to the staff within the Third Sector services they were attending. All data collection took place within the Mobile Dental Unit, which was a small confined space. Outside of the dental surgery section of the Unit there was a waiting area with enough space for approximately two people—any more than two and it began to feel crowded. This meant that it was not the most appropriate place for impromptu oral health advice or longer discussions about oral health with service users.

The observations at the Mobile Dental Unit (MDU) highlighted an additional barrier to the working alliance between the oral health practitioners and the service users—that there are risks involved in delivering Smile4life and that the service users can be unpredictable and occasionally violent. On a number of occasions, disruptive service users were observed barging into the Unit, demanding to be seen by a dentist. In these instances, the oral health practitioner was the one who acted as a gatekeeper, preventing the service users from accessing the dental surgery section of the Unit.

> "When I was there today two service users opened the MDU door from the outside and barged in"
>
> (Observation 3)

> "When I arrived there were two women outside the front door (of the MDU) shouting."
>
> (Observation 4)

Perceptions of there being risks associated with Smile4life delivery were strengthened by the repeated use of safety measures, such as alarms or radios, in the services visited while observing the oral health practitioners. In most instances, these devices were given to the oral health practitioner by the Third Sector staff before they proceeded to interact with service users—the researcher never observed an emergency alarm or radio being used. Indeed, it became apparent that the oral health practitioners did not feel they were at risk, despite Practitioner 1 having a good reason to be concerned about her safety. She told the researcher that on a previous visit to a drop-in she had been bitten on the hand by a service user, while she had been discussing oral health with him. This event was then reported to Datix, the NHS's incident reporting tool. However, when she saw that he was present at the session we were attending, she did not avoid him and spoke with him again. At the same session, Practitioner 1 had warned the researcher beforehand to be careful about her handbag, because some of the service users had been known to steal.

3.1.2. Enablers

It became clear that there were two key factors in overcoming these barriers and enabling a successful working alliance to be formed between the oral health practitioners and the service users: the skills and attitudes of the oral health practitioners and the use of incentives.

With regard to the oral health practitioners themselves, the researcher observed that they needed to be confident, and in some respects, fearless. Indeed, the field notes frequently reflect this:

> "Working in the mobile dental unit would not be for everyone—you need to be confident and thick-skinned"
>
> (Observation 3)

> "Practitioner 1 is confident and appears quite fearless, putting up with language/behaviour that would not be tolerated in a normal clinic."
>
> (Observation 6)

> "I get the impression that Practitioner 4 and the other practitioners I have observed . . . do not see the risk involved in their job, or they just see it as part of the job . . . it is also possible that after a while doing this kind of work they stop seeing it as risky"
>
> (Observation 9)

It became apparent that working on Smile4life was not something that would suit everyone—the oral health practitioners themselves said as much.

> "The dental team spoke about how they felt that working in the MDU would not suit everyone"
>
> (Observation 3)

> "I believe that not everyone is suited to doing Practitioner 1's job—personality aside, you need to be fast-thinking, tough-skinned, a bit fearless, and approachable."
>
> (Observation 6)

In addition to confidence, the oral health practitioners also had to be flexible in their interactions with service users, in particular, tolerating disruptive behaviour, for a working alliance to be sustained. In Board 1, the oral health practitioner, and the dentist and dental nurse who worked in the Mobile Dental Unit, described some service users as being disruptive, trying to flirt with them and one man who had taken off his t-shirt to show them his tattoos. Other service users swore or used offensive language. The oral health practitioners admitted that they tolerated this kind of behaviour from the patients they saw in the MDU, but would not normally do so, with patients they saw in their usual clinics. In the case where the patient was flirting and removing his clothes, they did not seem fazed by this. It became apparent over the course of the observation sessions that the success of engagement attempts was closely associated with the individual oral health practitioner, and their personality, experience, communication skills and how they perceived their job role and responsibilities.

From this, it appears that, for the oral health practitioner to be successful in implementing Smile4life, they needed to be flexible, not just in their working hours (e.g., working in the evenings) but also in tolerating disruptive behaviours from patients, while remaining non-judgmental and not taking undue risks. They must tailor their approach to the needs of the individual service user.

> "Practitioner 1 is very experienced and upfront with all service users—not visibly fazed by service users' admissions or behaviours"
>
> (Observation 1)

> "The MDU dentist admitted that she is aware that she acts differently with patients in the MDU than she would with regular patients—she is not as formal, more likely to speak to them in the same way they speak to her . . . she is quite matter-of-fact"
>
> (Observation 3)

Furthermore, the researcher observed that the oral health practitioners have to be very sensitive and empathetic, to strengthen the working alliance—often service users will share information about their lives, and their past experiences, and practitioners must listen and respond appropriately. The oral health practitioners at the MDU were observed speaking affectionately about long-term patients, and remembering everyone's names. Others were observed tailoring their advice to the needs of the service users, and letting service users tell their stories about their lives, occasionally attempting to bring the conversation back to oral health. In some instances, the oral health practitioner would share their own life experiences if it was related to the topics that were being discussed:

> "When a service user said he found it difficult to stop smoking, Practitioner 1 admitted that she was an ex-smoker, and explained that she still feels tempted"
>
> *(Observation 1)*

The oral health practitioner in Board 3 demonstrated on numerous occasions that she was willing to go the extra mile for the service users she sees. These extra tasks that she does are not because she has been asked to by her managers, but because she cares about the service users, and wants to offer them the best service she can.

> "To me it seems that Practitioner 4 goes above and beyond for the service users she sees. She will offer to phone and make appointments, sends them reminders the day before (even on her day off) and she will even take them to an appointment. It's clear that she cares if they attend or not—she mentioned that she has asked some practices to waive fines, and clearly advocates for the service users when necessary."
>
> *(Observation 8)*

Incentives were also used, to encourage service users to engage with the oral health practitioners, aiding in the development and maintenance of the working alliance. These were predominantly toothbrush and toothpaste packs, but in some NHS Boards could also be free samples of a wider range of toothpastes (e.g., Oral-B or Corsodyl), denture-care packs, or toothbrush cases. Indeed, service users were always eager to get the free samples of the branded toothpastes, compared to the more basic NHS-provided packs. These incentives often acted as an icebreaker, particularly in locations where the oral health practitioner had to approach service users to see if they were interested in discussing oral health, rather than interested service users approaching them. In some instances, when a wide range of resources were available, they were also an opportunity for the oral health practitioners to find out more about the service users oral health—they could ask questions under the pretence of ensuring they gave them the most appropriate product. For example:

> "Practitioner 1 would take the time to find free samples that would be specific to the service user, e.g., Corsodyl toothpaste for people with bleeding gums, or denture care items"
>
> *(Observation 1)*

3.2. Alliance 2: Oral Health Practitioners and Third Sector Staff

While considering Alliance 1, it became apparent that Smile4life delivery may be reduced if there is no alliance between the oral health practitioners and the Third Sector staff. The cooperation of the Third Sector staff is crucial as they allow the oral health practitioner access to their service and their service users. For example, they can choose to promote Smile4life and visits from the oral health practitioner or do nothing to encourage service users to be interested in their oral health. In the observations, the Third Sector staff often acted as a barrier to alliances forming between them and the oral health practitioners, as well as between the oral health practitioners and the service users. Alternatively, in one NHS Board, the oral health practitioners themselves were a barrier to a working alliance with local Third Sector staff. These barriers are discussed in more depth below.

3.2.1. Barriers

In Board 1, there was no observed working alliance between the oral health practitioners, service users or Third Sector staff. Unlike the more pro-active oral health practitioners observed in the other Boards, in Board 1, the oral health practitioners did not approach service users—they offered a mobile dental unit and if any service user was interested in getting treatment they had to approach the unit.

> "Practitioner 3 did not really interact with service users beyond telling them if they can be seen by the dentist, or making general conversation. She would encourage people to wait in the drop-in rather than in the MDU before their treatment"
>
> *(Observation 3)*

> "The oral health team do not seem bothered to recruit any patients, even if that means sitting waiting with nothing to do—the feeling seems to be that if a patient wants to be seen then they will come to the MDU."
>
> (Observation 4)

In the other two NHS Boards, in most instances, the oral health practitioner was reliant on the Third Sector staff at the organisations to promote and advertise the oral health visits, e.g., by putting up posters, flyers, or announcing the visit over the overhead speaker. However, this was often not the case:

> "In all three establishments today, staff did not seem well prepared for Practitioner 2's visit—her poster was only displayed in one of them, and they had not spoken to their service users about her visit ... In one place, the room we were offered was in the staff area, so there would never be any passing service users"
>
> (Observation 2)

This excerpt from the field notes highlights the extent to which the oral health practitioner is at the mercy of the Third Sector staff—during that observation, the oral health practitioner visited three services and only spoke to one service user. At the first service, the oral health practitioner had been advised to attend at a time when there were no service users awake; at the second, the oral health practitioner was given a room to use which was a meeting room in the staff area. There was also no attempt by Third Sector staff at any of the three locations to let their service users know that Practitioner 2 was available to talk to. This suggests that, if the oral health practitioner does not know the staff that well, they are not motivated to prioritise her requests or to put up her posters. Similarly, if they do not understand the importance of oral health then they would be unlikely to encourage their service users to care about their oral health.

3.2.2. Enablers

Despite the barriers discussed above, any potential alliance between the oral health practitioner and the Third Sector staff was dependent on both parties engaging with each other. While the previous example demonstrated that, when the Third Sector staff do not help the oral health practitioners, Smile4life cannot be delivered and it is the responsibility of the oral health practitioner to attempt to establish a relationship in the first instance. As with forming an alliance with service users, the oral health practitioners were themselves an enabler to forming relationships with the Third Sector staff.

> "it is clear that Practitioner 1 works hard at maintaining strong relationships with staff at these locations ... she makes a point of visiting every 6 weeks and reminds them the day before that she will be visiting."
>
> (Observation 1)

> "Practitioner 1 clearly has a good relationship with the staff ... she told me that 'keeping the staff sweet' is a major part of her role and really helps with building rapport"
>
> (Observation 7)

As with service users, incentives also aided in the formation of an alliance with the Third Sector staff—Practitioner 1 said as much when she told the researcher that she needed to "keep the staff sweet" so would purposively keep two packs of PolyGrip aside for one member of staff in particular (Observation 7).

3.3. Alliance 3: Third Sector Staff and Service Users

The third alliance that exists between the three key parties involved in Smile4life is the one between the Third Sector staff and the service users. However, interactions between the Third Sector staff and the service users were not observed during the present study as the oral health practitioners were the focus of the participant observation—this, therefore, represents a limitation with regard to dental care policy. The need remains to conduct additional studies to confirm this process to provide dental care for people experiencing homelessness.

4. Discussion

The findings from the observation sessions suggest that key factors in the delivery of Smile4life are the working alliances among the oral health practitioners, the Third Sector staff and the service users.

Within this triad, there are three key alliances: (1) oral health practitioners and service users; (2) oral health practitioners and Third Sector staff; and (3) Third Sector staff and service users. When there are strong working alliances, the Third Sector staff can promote and signpost to the oral health practitioner, who in turn can engage directly with service users about their oral health.

With regard to Simmel's work concerning coalitions within a triad, in an ideal Smile4life scenario, the Third Sector staff would act as a "non-partisan", facilitating a connection between the oral health practitioner and the service users [30]. Indeed, this was the case in the more successful interactions that were observed, However, it is apparent from the observation data that this was not always the case: while not necessarily partisan, it would appear that some Third Sector staff were indifferent about oral health. In these instances, it is possible that the Third Sector staff interpreted the oral health practitioners as intruders, disturbing their existing dyadic relationship with their service users, or potentially excluding them from the triad. Due to this possible interpretation, in many cases, it is the Third Sector staff that hold the power within the triad—they can control access to the service and the service users, essentially acting as gatekeepers to protect the service users from what they may perceive as a threat, i.e., the "tertius gaudens" scenario as described by Simmel [30].

However, in instances where the Third Sector staff are helpful—and perhaps the communication between parties is more effective—there can still be the issue of disinterested or disruptive service users. In these cases, the power distribution shifts and it is the service users that hold the power—it is up to them if they are receptive to Smile4life, or whether they will be rude and disinterested in what the oral health practitioner has to say. For example, in instances such as those observed in Boards 1 and 2, the service users demonstrated their power by being disruptive or argumentative with the oral health practitioners, e.g., arguing about fluoride.

Interestingly, in both scenarios, the oral health practitioners are powerless. Indeed, in many respects, they *are* intruders, or outsiders, attempting to infiltrate the service where the Third Sector staff and the service users are based. In this respect, when the oral health practitioner enters, they allow a majority to form, i.e., two against one [29]. Caplow examined the power dynamics and coalitions present in three-person groups and considered there to be eight types of coalition, dependent on the power held by each of the three parties, e.g., A = B = C, where all parties are equal; or A < B, B = C, where B and C have equal power, which is greater than that of A—this could be said to be the case when oral health practitioners are seen as intruding upon the existing alliance of the Third Sector staff and the service users [31].

However, due to the scope of the research and the focus on the oral health practitioners, it was not possible to observe Alliance 3, and therefore not possible to fully explore the different power dynamics present in the three-party group. This is a limitation of this research, and a potential topic for future studies in this area. Observing the relationship between the Third Sector staff and the service users would reveal if oral health is considered a priority for these individuals, particularly in the absence of the oral health practitioners. It would also aid in a deeper understanding of how the triadic working alliance operates, and if the entrance of the oral health practitioners is truly seen as an intrusion, forcing the three-person group into "a pair and an other", with the oral health practitioner being the "other" [32] (p. 351) [30].

There are also limitations associated with participant observation as a data collection tool. While it allows the researcher to gain first-hand experience of the topic being studied, it is not repeatable, and is dependent on the researcher's interpretations of what is being observed [33]. It is also time-consuming, requiring the researcher to spend long periods with the participants being observed [22]. However, despite these limitations, it was an appropriate tool for this study, as it allowed the authors to immerse themselves in the working lives of the oral health practitioners, which would not necessarily have been possible with other data collection methods, e.g., interviews. While it was time-consuming, this provided the "time to develop an intuitive feel for the particular system studied" [33] (p. 37).

While the observations concerned the delivery of the Smile4life intervention and the relationships between oral health practitioners, homeless service users and Third Sector staff, it is possible that the results could be generalisable to any situation where oral health is being delivered to an excluded or vulnerable population, such as adults with learning disabilities. Many of the barriers faced by the oral health practitioners could be considered organisational barriers, which are not specific to the homelessness context (e.g., uncooperative Third Sector staff and lack of access to service users/patients). Similarly, the factors identified as enablers to the alliances discussed above (e.g., the skills and attitude of the oral health practitioners) would be beneficial to any oral health practitioner attempting to forge a good working relationship with any patients or organisations, not just within homelessness.

With regard to recommendations for the continued delivery of the Smile4life intervention, based on the observations, it would appear that there needs to be a strengthened relationship—or alliance—between the oral health practitioners and the Third Sector staff. Specifically, there should be more awareness raising about the benefits of Smile4life and what the oral health practitioners are attempting to do when they visit a Third Sector organisation. This would potentially overcome the issue of the location or physical space the oral health practitioner is given to deliver Smile4life. Additional buy-in from the Third Sector could also facilitate improved access to the service users, if the Third Sector staff see the importance of oral health and encourage their service users to see the oral health practitioner. However, it must be acknowledged that some barriers experienced by the oral health practitioners are organisational issues, such as staffing within the Third Sector organisation, and as such are not straightforward to overcome. In addition, it would be necessary to investigate the barriers and enablers in more detail, to establish what the oral health practitioners themselves think of their experiences and their role in delivering Smile4life, before any changes are recommended regarding the delivery of Smile4life.

5. Conclusions

The observation sessions have demonstrated how Smile4life is implemented in three different NHS Boards across Scotland, and highlighted the variations in practitioners' approaches to their Smile4life-related work. Furthermore, they revealed the three key working alliances that exist among the oral health practitioners, the Third Sector staff and the service users. By referring to theories of triadic coalitions, it was possible to infer the types of relationships that exist within the triad, and the power dynamics that exist within these relationships. To successfully deliver Smile4life to service users, all parties in the triad must work together, and each of the three key alliances must be strong. There can be no Alliance 1 if Alliances 2 and 3 do not already exist. In addition, there were many factors that influenced these alliances, and these acted as barriers and enablers to strong and beneficial relationships.

Author Contributions: This work forms part of L.B.'s doctoral research and is taken from her thesis. Conceptualisation, L.B.; Formal analysis, L.B.; Investigation, L.B.; Methodology, L.B.; Supervision, I.A., G.H., A.R. and R.F.; Visualisation, L.B.; Writing—original draft, L.B.; and Writing—review and editing, L.B., I.A., G.H., A.R. and R.F.

Funding: The Smile4life programme was funded by the Scottish Government and National Health Service Boards (grant number: 121.80.4497).

Acknowledgments: We are grateful to the NHS practitioners for taking part in this research.

Conflicts of Interest: The authors declare no conflict of interest.

References

1. Somerville, P. Understanding homelessness. *Hous. Theory Soc.* **2013**, *30*, 384–415. [CrossRef]
2. Collins, J. Characterising Homeless People in Scotland: Can Oral Health, Health and Psychosocial Wellbeing Enhance the ETHOS Typology of Homelessness. Ph.D. Thesis, University of Dundee, Dundee, Scotland, 2012.
3. Scottish Government. *Homelessness in Scotland: 2015–16*; Scottish Government: Edinburgh, Scotland, 2016.
4. Fitzpatrick, S.; Johnsen, S.; White, M. Multiple Exclusion Homelessness in the UK: Key patterns and intersections. *Soc. Policy Soc.* **2011**, *10*, 501–512. [CrossRef]
5. Collins, J.; Freeman, R. Homeless in North and West Belfast: An oral health needs assessment. *Br. Dent. J.* **2007**, *202*, E31. [CrossRef] [PubMed]
6. Chi, D.; Milgrom, P. The oral health of homeless adolescents and young adults and determinants of oral health: Preliminary findings. *Spec. Care Dent.* **2008**, *28*, 237–242. [CrossRef] [PubMed]
7. Figueiredo, R.L.F.; Hwang, S.W.; Quiñonez, C. Dental health of homeless adults in Toronto, Canada. *J. Public Health Dent.* **2013**, *73*, 74–78. [CrossRef] [PubMed]
8. NHS Health Scotland. *Inequality Briefing: Health and Homelessness*; NHS Health Scotland: Edinburgh, Scotland, 2016.
9. Groundswell. *Healthy Mouths: A Peer-Led Health Audit on the Oral Health of People Experiencing Homelessness*; Groundswell: London, UK, 2017.
10. Scottish Executive. *Health and Homelessness Standards*; Scottish Executive: Edinburgh, Scotland, 2005.
11. Scottish Executive. *An Action Plan for Improving Oral Health and Modernising NHS Dental Services*; Scottish Executive: Edinburgh, Scotland, 2005.
12. NHS Principles and Values. Available online: https://www.nhs.uk/using-the-nhs/about-the-nhs/principles-and-values/ (accessed on 31 October 2018).
13. Wanyonyi, K.L.; Themessl-Huber, M.; Humphris, G.; Freeman, R. A systematic review of meta-analysis of face-to-face communication of tailored health messages: Implications for practice. *Patient Educ. Couns.* **2011**, *85*, 348–355. [CrossRef] [PubMed]
14. Scottish Government. *National Oral Health Improvement Strategy for Priority Groups*; Scottish Government: Edinburgh, Scotland, 2012.
15. Coles, E.; Edwards, M.; Elliott, G.; Heffernan, A.; Moore, A.; Freeman, R. *Smile4life: The Oral Health of Homeless People in Scotland*; University of Dundee: Dundee, Scotland, 2011.
16. Freeman, R.; Coles, E.; Watt, C.; Edwards, M.; Jones, C. *Smile4life Guide for Trainers: Better Oral Care for Homeless People*; NHS Health Scotland: Edinburgh, Scotland, 2012.
17. Beaton, L.; Freeman, R. Oral health promotion and homelessness: A theory-based approach to understanding processes of implementation and adoption. *Health Educ. J.* **2016**, *75*, 184–197. [CrossRef]
18. Mays, N.; Pope, C. Observational methods in health care settings. *Br. Med. J.* **1995**, *311*, 182–184. [CrossRef]
19. Ekins, R. *Male Femaling: A Grounded Theory Approach to Cross-Dressing and Sex Changing*; Routledge: London, UK, 1997; ISBN 0415106249.
20. Scottish Government. *Operation of the Homeless Persons Legislation in Scotland*; Scottish Government: Edinburgh, Scotland, 2015.
21. Taylor-Powell, E.; Steele, S. *Collecting Evaluation Data: Direct Observation. Programme Development and Evaluation*; Cooperative Extension Publications: Madison, WI, USA, 1996.
22. Zhao, M.; Ji, Y. Challenges of introducing participant observation to community health research. *ISRN Nurs.* **2014**. [CrossRef] [PubMed]
23. Jorgensen, D.L. *Participant Observation: A methodology for Human Studies*; SAGE Publications Inc.: Thousand Oaks, CA, USA, 1989; ISBN 0803928777.
24. Elo, S.; Kyngäs, H. The qualitative content analysis process. *J. Adv. Nurs.* **2008**, *62*, 107–115. [CrossRef] [PubMed]
25. Silverman, D. *Interpreting Qualitative Data*, 4th ed.; SAGE Publications Ltd.: London, UK, 2011; ISBN 0857024213.

26. Birks, M.; Chapman, Y.; Francis, K. Memoing in qualitative research: Probing data and processes. *J. Res. Nurs.* **2008**, *13*, 68–75. [CrossRef]
27. Mayring, P. Qualitative Content Analysis. *Forum Qual. Soc. Res.* **2000**, *1*, 20.
28. Bordin, E.S. The generalisability of the psychoanalytic concept of the working alliance. *Psychother. Theory Res. Pract.* **1979**, *16*, 252–260. [CrossRef]
29. Hill, L.B.; McGrath, J.M. Communication within the triadic context: Intercultural prospects. *Intercult. Commun. Stud.* **2008**, *17*, 52–67.
30. Simmel, G. *The Sociology of Georg Simmel*; Wolff, K.H., Translator; Wolff, K.H., Ed.; Free Press: New York, NY, USA, 1950; ISBN 1296031292.
31. Caplow, T. Further development of a theory of coalitions in the triad. *Am. J. Sociol.* **1959**, *64*, 488–493. [CrossRef]
32. Mills, T.M. Power relations in three-person groups. *Am. Sociol. Rev.* **1953**, *18*, 351–357. [CrossRef]
33. Robinson, D.T.; Brown, D.G.; Parker, D.C.; Schreinemachers, P.; Janssen, M.A.; Huigen, M.; Wittmer, H.; Gotts, N.; Promburom, P.; Irwins, E.; et al. Comparison of empirical methods for building agent-based models in land use science. *J. Land Use Sci.* **2007**, *2*, 31–55. [CrossRef]

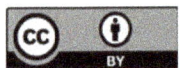

© 2018 by the authors. Licensee MDPI, Basel, Switzerland. This article is an open access article distributed under the terms and conditions of the Creative Commons Attribution (CC BY) license (http://creativecommons.org/licenses/by/4.0/).

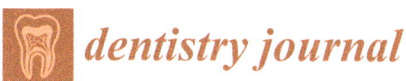

Article

Strengthening Social Interactions and Constructing New Oral Health and Health Knowledge: The Co-design, Implementation and Evaluation of A Pedagogical Workshop Program with and for Homeless Young People

Andrea Rodriguez *, Laura Beaton and Ruth Freeman *

Dental Health Services Research Unit, School of Dentistry, University of Dundee, Dundee DD1 4HN, UK; l.z.beaton@dundee.ac.uk
* Correspondence: a.rodriguez@dundee.ac.uk (A.R.); r.e.freeman@dundee.ac.uk (R.F.)

Received: 9 October 2018; Accepted: 17 January 2019; Published: 1 February 2019

Abstract: Young homeless people make up nearly one-third of those experiencing homelessness. The need to provide an educative approach, to strengthen social interacting, and construct new knowledge to increase social inclusivity, is required. The aim of this qualitative exploration was to use critical consciousness as an educative tool, to co-design, implement, and evaluate a series of oral health and health pedagogical workshops to strengthen social engagement and to construct new health knowledge, with, and for, homeless young people and their service providers. An action research design permitted the simultaneous development, implementation, and evaluation of the pedagogical workshop program. A Non-Governmental Organization (NGO), providing supported accommodation for young homeless people, acted as the partner organization. Thirteen young people and five staff members from this NGO participated and co-designed eight workshops. Qualitative data collection included unstructured post-intervention interviews together with verbatim quotes from the group discussions during the workshops and from the post-workshop questionnaires. The qualitative analysis was informed by content analysis to permit the emergence of key themes from the data. The two themes were: 1. 'trust building and collective engaging' and 2. 'constructing knowledge and developing skills'. Theme 1 highlighted engagement with the service provider, illustrating the transformation of the young people's relationships, strengthening of their social interacting, and enabling their critical reflexive thinking on sensitive issues present in the homelessness trajectory. Theme 2 illustrated the young people's ability to share, lend, and encode their new health information and convert it into an understandable and useable form. This new comprehension permitted their behavior change and social interaction. These findings provide an approach to increase young people's knowledge, health literacy, and strengthen their social interacting to support community action.

Keywords: pedagogical approaches; young people; homelessness; critical consciousness

1. Introduction

Recent news reports on young homeless people have put youth homelessness at center-stage. Research that was commissioned by the BBC showed that over 40% of young people sofa surfed with friends for long periods of time without seeking support from Local Authorities [1]. In Scotland, 28% of all homelessness applications were from people aged between 16 and 24 years [2]. The Scottish Government linked youth homelessness to social and health-related factors [2–5] and called for a joint and multiagency approach to tackle the health and social care challenges of young homeless people [6]. It has been shown that youth homelessness is caused by family and relationship break-down, exacerbated by youth unemployment, escalating rent costs, and overall benefit cuts [7]. The result has been poorer physical and mental health in young people experiencing homelessness [8,9]. Hence, youth homelessness has been identified as a serious and chronic social problem.

The Scottish Government developed a series of homelessness policies [10–14] that recognized the need for a holistic approach that not only address housing, but also other critical issues, such as physical and psychosocial needs, including the effects on mental health and oral health associated with being young and homeless. What brings all of these health aspects together is the common risk factor approach (CRFA) [15]. Oral health, in this regard, is included in the CRFA and allows dentistry and oral health promotion to be key features in addressing the social aspects of psychosocial health and wellbeing, i.e., low self-esteem, reduced employment opportunities, or isolation. Despite these policy recommendations and CFRA interventions to prevent and/or solve health and oral health problems, young people experiencing homelessness continued to experience limited access and engagement with health and social care services [16,17]. Within a lexicon of mistrust, negativity, perceived stigmatization, and acknowledged awkwardness, [18,19], significant communication barriers exist between those utilizing and those providing oral health, health, and social services. In their exploration of community health workers, Gale et al. [19] posed that the communication between health workers and clients was unusual, as their interactions were content and time-limited with none of the spontaneity of social interacting. They conceptualized this type of interaction as a 'synthetic social interaction', and while appropriate for health workers to communicate oral health and health service information, it inadvertently promoted a more paternalistic communication style, with a top-down approach that resulted in feelings of mistrust, stigma, and/or negativity in client groups. This work [19] questioned the approaches used and called for new creative and participative methods to engage with young people experiencing homelessness. There was a need to promote a more spontaneous and social interaction style that would permit the promotion of joint working and engagement between client and practitioner, ultimately to improve health, oral health, and psychosocial wellbeing.

Using an educational tool to facilitate this interaction would allow engagement and effective communication between participants. Thinking in this way, the issue of young people's apparent absence of motivation to engage with dental and health and social service practitioners, required reassessment. Rather, it was the intervention content, sometimes subject to a prejudicial judgment, together with a paternalistic style of interacting, which had the potential to exacerbate young people's fears of stigmatization and rejection. This was observed as a disinclination to engage with health and social care professionals. The need to provide an environment to enable collaborative working for increased wider health knowledge and service engagement appeared to be urgently required.

In order to achieve engagement with services providers, critical reflexion on aspects of their reality and spontaneous interaction would be necessary to work in a cooperative manner. For Wolfe et al. [20], working cooperatively means improved psychosocial and cognitive skills, which in turn increase health learning capacity: for Freeman [21], it is how the participants encode the received information, how they make the information their own, which paves the way for better health literacy: for Freire [22], it is the practice of dialogue that helps to form critical consciousness and critical attitudes for learning, critical thinking, and action, with the formation of new knowledge. The practice of dialogue on sensitive issues, between service-user and service provider, is thus central for the development of understandable forms of health information and new life choices. The dialogue in Freire's perspective is not just about expressing ideas from one individual to another, nor is it simply about exchanging ideas with others. The dialogue in Freire's perspective [23] is an act of existential creation. Adopting this co-design strategy, based on Freire's theoretical approach to nurture social interacting, would promote joint decision-making, strengthening social change, health literacy, and health information gain [15]. This would permit the health cognitions, health literacy, and numeracy needs of the young people experiencing homelessness to be acknowledged and managed.

In essence, what is suggested is a participatory approach that is underpinned by Freire's formulation [22,23] to increase critical consciousness about how current problems in society are perceived, to provoke critical attitudes on challenges that affect vulnerable and marginalized groups, and to promote communication for health learning capacity. Freire's approach analyses degrees of understanding of reality and its relation to socio-cultural conditioning. The critical consciousness is characterized by the depth with which it interprets current problems, characterized by the autonomous and committed thinking that leads to socio-political engagement. Freire's dialogic knowledge exchange procedure allows for the development of activities to encourage and support participants to bring their own knowledge and share their life experiences in order to make conscious choices of action. In this study, the workshop program on health promotion acted as a vehicle for this.

The importance of working in groups to debate and to increase awareness of current problems in the wider context, as highlighted by Freire [23], has been emphasized by Candau & Sacavino [24] through their pedagogical workshop framework. Their framework adopts principles of Freire's theoretical approach understanding this resource (in the form of workshops) as a tool to overcome feelings of passivity and powerlessness in the face of social problems that are experienced by vulnerable and marginalized groups. These authors, in alignment with Freire, state that it is often in the interaction with peers that identities, critical reflexion, and knowledge are strengthened and can be structured in actions that aim for transformation [24]. It would seem that the dialogue approach offered by the workshop program would improve understanding of the links between health and homelessness journeys, health literacy, and the quality of interactions and engagement between excluded young people and health and social care practitioners. On this basis, will the use of pedagogical workshops act to stimulate reflection towards a conscious practice, for the development of the critical spirit, inciting the recognition of its individual and collective story, having, as a consequence, the perspective of changing structures that generates abrupt social inequalities?

Rodriguez's previous research with vulnerable youths in Brazil was also built around this framework to conduct community-based interventions, including their development and implementation simultaneously [25,26]. Following Freire and Rodriguez, this study adopted the view that there must be a deep understanding of the young persons' life experiences, as a foundation to develop trust, enables engagement, mutual learning, and knowledge construction. For Rodriguez the core element of enabling engagement and strengthening of social change for excluded youths is the ability of the health and/or social care professional to respond sensitively to 'the vulnerable young person's health and psychosocial needs in the face of marginalization and exclusion' [25]. In order to promote sensitivity and inclusion, it is necessary to have a forum that enables a person-centered approach and thereby shifts communication from synthetic to spontaneous social interacting, to support a process of building trust, new knowledge, the exploration of life experiences, and current life circumstances.

We argue that co-designed interventions that adopt the above strategy [22,24], together with Rodriguez's formulation [25,26] of shared working to strengthen social change, will ensure that their oral health and health issues will be sensitively explored. A two-pronged approach of (i) an understanding of communication and health interventions that divide, stigmatize, and label youth experiencing homelessness and (ii) the reflection and the dialogue between participants, has the potential for success. Using a pedagogical workshop strategy provides a safe space; permits young and homeless people to speak of their oral health and health concerns; and, allows for a critical reflection upon their life circumstances and enables engagement with practitioners. Therefore, the aim of this qualitative exploration was to use critical consciousness [22,23] as an educative tool, to co-design, implement, and evaluate a series of oral health and health workshops to strengthen social engagement and construct new health knowledge, with, and for, young people experiencing homeless.

2. Materials and Methods

The method used here to promote the active participation of a Non-Governmental Organization (NGO), practitioners, and young people was the dialogical approach proposed by Freire [22].

2.1. Theoretical Underpinning of the Pedagogical Workshop Program

In order to achieve successful engagement, participation and co-design, it is necessary to ensure that [i] the NGOs assisting in designing and hosting the intervention; [ii] the service providers co-delivering the activities; and, [iii] service users receiving an intervention in which their views and life experiences are integrated and they can play an active role within the whole developmental process [27].

2.2. Design

This qualitative exploration used an action research design to permit the simultaneous development, implementation, and evaluation of the pedagogical workshop program [28].

2.3. Procedure

2.3.1. Research Context

The NGO was identified for the pedagogical workshop program specifically because of the well-known work with young people aged between 16 and 24 years who were homeless. Their remit was to 'advise, educate and support young people' and 'to enable them to build life skills and the resources required to make a positive and healthy transition to adulthood' [29].

2.3.2. Gathering the Participants: The Sample

Initially, a convenience sample of NGO managers, and their front-line staff were invited to participate. The group was recruited by the principal investigator (PI) through previous contact with the NGO partner as a first phase of the development work (Table 1). Five of the NGO's staff members also participated in the eight workshops and evaluation (Table 1).

Table 1. Pedagogical workshop development.

Developmental Phase	Procedure	Outcomes
Phase 1	The selection of a key NGO supporting youth homeless in Scotland through a preliminary mapping of homelessness services and organizations. A series of meetings between the PI with staff members of the NGO and with youth homeless living in temporary accommodations. Identification of the main topics to be covered through the workshops as agreed by all participants. Co-design and delivery of the workshops.	An initial package of four workshops planned as requested by staff members and the young people, delivered and evaluated. Topics: [i] Oral health, [ii] Mental health, [iii] Education & the future, [iv] Stigma Planning of the workshops involved a multidisciplinary collaboration between the PI with one NHS Board and one NGO to provide expert knowledge on the evidence-base and current guidance on oral health and mental health. Evaluation by direct observation on participants' feedback and group discussion during the workshops, and post-workshop questionnaires.
Phase 2	Following the same participative approach, the feedback received following Phase 1 was positive, and the young people requested further workshops. Meetings with young people were convened to discuss openly and using critical consciousness, to identify the additional workshop topics regarding the workshop package 2. Co-design and delivery of the workshops.	A second package of workshops was planned, delivered and evaluated following the same procedure as in Phase 1. Topics requested by the young people: [i] Homeless trajectory, [ii] Substance misuse, [iii] Resilience, [iv] Healthy eating Planning of the workshops again involved a multidisciplinary collaboration between the PI with one NHS Board and one NGO to provide expert knowledge on the evidence-base and current guidance on substance use, resilience, and healthy eating.

Table 1. *Cont.*

Developmental Phase	Procedure	Outcomes
Phase 3	Semi-structured interviews with all participants to explore key issues raised during the workshops including perceptions of the efficacy and appropriateness of using pedagogical workshops to explore the life experiences, views and opinions of the young people	Identification of key issues and perceptions of efficacy and appropriateness of workshops.

A purposive and non-probability sample of young people who were living in temporary and supportive accommodations provided by the NGO was invited to participate: their recruitment was facilitated by staff members who were working directly with them. The NGO staff were informed of the voluntary nature of the young person's participation. The invitation to take part in the study was provided initially in the form of a poster advertisement, placed in common areas of passage of young people, inviting those interested to contact staff members. Secondly, information sheets were provided to those who requested additional information. After a cooling off period of a month, the young people who had decided to participate completed the consent form with the PI. A total of 13 young people took part in the workshop program and evaluation (Table 1).

2.3.3. Pedagogical Workshop Program: Phases of Development

Phase 1: A series of meetings took place between the PI and managers, staff members of the NGO, and young homeless people living in temporary accommodation, with the intention of co-designing the content and delivery of the workshops. In these three initial meetings, an identification of four main topics on health promotion to be covered through the workshops was agreed by all participants. The meetings, in phase 1, guaranteed that mutual trust was built between the PI and the participants providing the foundation for an open exploration of key health and social concerns of young people experiencing homeless. Having jointly identified and selected key health promotion topics for the first workshops, the PI engaged with one NHS Board and one NGO to ensure that the information provided at the workshops was evidence-practice based and complied with current guidance. The first package of workshops (four) was then jointly planned, delivered, and evaluated through direct observation [30] during the workshops, and with post-questionnaires given to participants and staff members. This package of workshops was delivered by the PI with the assistance of an oral health promoter from the NHS Board and a research assistant.

Phase 2: This phase adopted a similar participatory approach as in Phase 1. Following completion of the first four workshops, the NGO and young participants required one more package of workshops. Discussion groups were conducted with all participants, and in particular the young people, to inform a second phase of workshop development. Phase 2 was characterized by an open discussion on the young participants' additional concerns and joint workshops' planning. Four additional concerns were identified by the homeless youth and staff members. The PI, as mentioned above, repeated the process implemented in Phase 1—once all the workshops' content had been agreed with all participants, one key NHS Board and one NGO were involved to contribute to the health-related information provided and confirmed that it was supported by recent literature. The second package of workshops (four) were planned, delivered, and evaluated using the same format as mentioned in Phase 1 (Table 1).

Phase 3: This phase formed part of the evaluation of the pedagogical workshop program and involved semi-structured interviews with some of the participants (Table 1).

The structure of the pedagogical workshop program is described below. It used critical consciousness as an educative tool to support awareness of self-knowledge, critical thinking, and co-construction of consensus, and a joint action plan for behavior change.

2.4. Pedagogical Workshop Program Structure and Timing

The structure and format of the workshops used Candau and Sacavino's framework [24] with some additions and adaptations to match and reflect the life experiences of the young homeless participants. A range of creative approaches to engage with the participants, and to accommodate their different learning styles, was incorporated into the workshops. Therefore, the Candau and Sacavino's framework [24] was not only linked with the Freire's theoretical position of 'tuning into the other's universe', but it also provided a means for its operationalization in the workshop setting. The workshops were undertaken in small groups following Freire's approach to facilitate the discussion of sensitive issues, and used blended learning strategies. Therefore, spontaneous social interactions were fostered in the workshops by promoting lively interaction, using art, drama, music, films, photographs, popular magazines, and any form of communication that would permit the participants to raise their voices and to express their views (Table 2). These tables show the content of each of the eight workshops, together with a description of their implementation.

Table 2. Content and implementation of co-designed workshops 1–8.

Workshop 1. Oral health	Exploration of group perceptions of oral health, fears and barriers to accessing dental treatment emerged. A spontaneous discussion of the psychosocial effects of poor oral health on self-esteem, social interaction, and employability occurred. Common and divergent experiences were then identified and built into collective strategies to achieve good oral health as a way to improve other aspects of life.
Workshop 2. Mental health	[Part 1] Exploration of group perceptions of wellbeing and mental health; health information on different mental health problems and their causes; treatments available; role of practitioners, friends and family to tackle mental health problem. [Part 2] Sensitive discussions of relationship breakdown as a cause of mental health problems among young people; sharing of life experiences with family members and/or partners; the group discussed how to improve communication; how to manage conflicts, differing beliefs and world views; consensus of how these factors can affected their well-being and mental health.
Workshop 3. Education & the future	[Part 1] The participants were asked to identify and discuss different levels of knowledge in their lives built from both formal education (e.g., courses, college or university) and life experience; the recognition that both types of learning are important and serve the context required. [Part 2] Discussion of aspirations for the future. To visualise this future the participants built a collage to express a life project involving and promoting their health and wellbeing. [Part 3] Identification of feelings coming with the life planning exercise and an exploration of how they would make healthier choices for a better future.
Workshop 4. Stigma	The aim of this workshop was to continue to humanise the gaze and to enable participants to discuss the meaning and process of the construction of stigma against groups in society and especially youth homelessness. Using favelas in Brazil and their youth residents as an example of a stigmatized group, the participants felt comfortable to bring their own experiences of bias and stigma and the agreed strategies they would use to deal with discrimination. The participants were invited to create a campaign against prejudice, stigma and discrimination towards homelessness.
Workshop 5. Homeless trajectory	Discussions around participants' definitions of being young and their homelessness journey; exploration of the positive/negative aspects of this period of their lives; identifying routes that lead to their homelessness. The group was invited to engage individually and/or as a group in activities to produce a consensus outcome using diverse and creative ways of expression to translate this knowledge into an action plan for their lives.
Workshop 6. Substance misuse	Increased participants' awareness and knowledge of substance misuse; focussing on the increased use of New Psychoactive Substances (NPS), by young people; exploration of their reasons for becoming involved in drug use; participants' consensus of how to deal with drug use and how to overcome involvement.
Workshop 7. Resilience	Discussion of the meaning of resilience as the capacity to adapt and overcome risk and adversity; exploration of how they may become more resilient; learning of life skills and strategies to build their strength when going through a difficult time. Through the identification of positive thoughts that lead to their social change and negative thoughts that hold them back, the participants worked on the construction of their resilience, their life goals for future planning and the different steps necessary to achieve these goals (an action plan).
Workshop 8. Health eating	Discussion of the role of food in people's daily lives beyond the survival aspect; raising awareness and understanding of food as a way to [1] encourage social interaction, [2] break cultural and social barriers, [3] engage with people, [4] increase health literacy and [5] promote wellbeing. The participants reflected upon health eating and the effect of their position and social inequalities as the main reason why people living in poverty do not eat healthy food. This provided the basis for a co-construction of knowledge and an action plan for healthy eating.

The workshops were held and incorporated into the routine activities that were already in place at the NGO partner and at a time suggested by the NGO managers to meet participants' availability. The entire workshop program (development, implementation, and evaluation) ran over a 10-month period and each workshop lasted for two hours.

2.5. Workshop Structure

(1) Shared meal: On arrival, and for the first 30 minutes of each the workshop, the NGO provided a meal for the young people. This meal was shared between the participants and the workshop facilitators and started a process of mutual trust and interaction, as proposed by Freire [19,20].

(2) Introduction: Icebreaker activities were introduced to acquaint the participants with one another, to engender a relaxed atmosphere, reduce barriers, and enable spontaneous interaction and discussion. The ice-breaker activities thus provoked openness within an informal learning environment. In this way, the spontaneity of the interaction was fostered to enable critical reflection, as described by Freire.

(3) Increasing awareness: During the workshops, the PI and the workshop facilitators captured the different concerns, knowledge, and life experiences of each participant. This was a crucial moment because what was captured from the participants' narratives informed the content to be explored later in the workshop. Following Freire's formulation, the participants involved were invited by the PI to share their own perceptions, knowledge, and experiences instead of receiving health advice in a more traditional format of a health promotion session. In doing this, there was a change in the perspective of learning based not only in passing or transmitting new information and knowledge, but also putting the participants at the centre of their learning process [22].

(4) Deepening and reflection: The shared views and experiences of young participants during the workshops was creatively combined into a cohesive whole and conveyed as 'new information'. The presentation of the 'new information' allowed a shift in awareness, an appreciation that they were not alone in their experiences and furthered a deeper critical reflection proposed by the topic(s) discussed. This step in the workshop addressed Freire's approach [23] to enable participants to explore their society and critically question key issues, identifying and making explicit their understanding of the nature of their past and present social situations to develop increased capacity for choice.

(5) Co-construction and synthesis: In order to reach a level of consensus among the participants and to enable them to take ownership of their own and 'new information', it was necessary for participants to continue the discursive process by facilitating the expression of their own opinions, views, and thoughts. This process enabled each aspect or point of view to be synthesized into a co-constructed knowledge base by engaging the group in diverse and creative debate and activities. This produced a new personal knowledge consensus to be translated into key information and insights for use in the future. This critical consciousness and the confrontation of their current life circumstances allowed for them to reflect on self-esteem, feelings of being stigmatized, their responsibilities, and roles to achieve social transformation [23].

(6) Group agreement and workshop close: The aim of the closure of the workshop was to invite participants to explain individually how their increased awareness, reflections, new personal knowledge, and insights, which were explored during the workshop, would be incorporated into their lives and daily routines. This encouraged the participants to translate their personal commitments into a group's action plan to support behavior change. Therefore, this last moment of the workshop illustrates Freire's proposition [22] that in consequence of a critical consciousness, a critical attitude can be formed toward healthier life choices.

2.6. Qualitative Data and Analysis

The intervention was evaluated using a qualitative methodology. The qualitative data included, for this purpose, direct observation and recorded discussions during the workshops, post-workshop in-depth interviews, and verbatim comments from the post-workshop questionnaires. During the workshops and the post-workshop interviews, the participants were invited to speak about the workshop experience and/or anything they wished to. They could stop talking when they wanted and could bring the interview to an end when they felt it was the right time. All of the workshops and interviews data were transcribed and subjected to content analysis [31].

Content analysis allows the transcribed data to be explored meticulously, line-by-line to discover categories, themes, and concepts [31]. The analysis, therefore, starts with exact and thorough line-by-line coding to identify categories and themes. The coding went beyond a simple description of the data context and therefore when an interesting idea/incident was noted this was catalogued to allow for a subsequent category to emerge. After the researchers independently examined the data they met together to discuss their categories and themes. When a disagreement occurred further discussions ensured that a consensus was reached and that the data were trustworthy.

2.7. Ethical Considerations

Ethical approval was obtained from the Research Ethics Committee at the University of Dundee (UREC 15149). Poster information and participant information sheets were provided, and consent forms were required to be completed prior to taking part in the workshops and post-workshop interviews (see ii). All of the data were anonymized and confidentiality ensured.

3. Results

Demographic Profile of the Participants

Thirteen young people (YP) participated in the workshops; eight were female and five were male. The sample was aged between 18 and 22 years. Five NGO practitioners participated in the workshops. Two were male and three were female. All of the young people (YP) and the NGO staff members (SM) contributed to the qualitative data presented.

The qualitative findings are described below. The presentation of the themes and their behavioral descriptors provide an illustration of how critical consciousness in the form of educational workshops may be developed and implemented for and with young people to promote health and psychosocial wellbeing.

Theme 1: Trust building and collective engaging

The first theme to emerge was 'trust building and collective engaging'. People need to feel safe in order to share their views and experiences. Trust building and collective engaging was characterized by open discussion, non-judgmental attitudes from the researcher and participants, liveliness, spontaneity, hearing and 'sharing experiences', thinking about life and current life circumstances, and deeper discussion of sensitive issues to achieve better health and well-being. The behavioral features of trust building and collective engaging were categorized as spontaneous social interacting and context enabling. Spontaneous social interacting reflected the motivation to share experiences and feelings in a trustful environment, and it became apparent that it supported the strengthening of the relationship between the young people themselves and with the practitioners. The following comments from the post-questionnaires are illustrative: 'What I most liked was to see the interaction between them, young people being comfortable about sharing experiences'. (SM 4); 'the best part of the workshop was the social discussion, really good fun' (YP 3); 'It was an informal chat' (YP 4); 'I could talk about normal life, issues related to me' (YP 5); and, 'We need to have more spaces like this to talk about life really helpful' (YP 7).

Context enabling described spontaneous social interaction among the young people. Direct observation, post-questionnaires, and interviews captured their perceptions about the workshops after each session. The workshops were seen as promoting an 'informal atmosphere', a 'welcoming and friendly environment', and a 'safe space' to share feelings, thoughts, beliefs, and experiences 'without judgment'. A staff member highlighted that the workshops created more opportunities for young people to express their lived experiences that otherwise might not have been revealed in a one-to-one session with the NGO staff:

"A young woman who attended the workshop around mental health, she was very vocal about her own experience of how mental health has been for her. She's not somebody that normally expresses much in a group, she's quite a private person, so I thought it took quite a lot for her to open up, to trust, but I also appreciate the fact that she felt she was in a really good space that she could share that experience with the others and I felt that was really valuable for the rest of the group to hear that. I think this activity [the workshops] encourages people to talk about their own experiences ". (SM 1).

The quote above suggests that the participants of the workshops were able to reveal difficult situations to their peers in the context of the group, because they felt that they were in a safe space to do so and, as these participants had a positive reception, this helped them to re-signify such experiences internally in a movement to overcome them.

An integral part of 'context enabling' was observed as the PI's attention to the participants' feedback during the process of the workshop program delivery, which promoted flexibility to change and to adapt the group activities to encourage the young people to participate, as illustrated by the comment of this staff member:

"I do want to say that I appreciate the way you [PI] tailored the sessions in response to the feedback that you got each session... and the way that you managed to structure the workshops so that there was more discussion and more interactivity". (SM 2)

The important behavioral aspects of trust building and collective engaging were spontaneous social interacting and context enabling and it was possible to conceptualize this theme and its behavioral dimensions as providing the ambiance for critical reflexive thinking [22]. To facilitate critical reflexive thinking there must be trust between all of the participants involved (i.e., context enabling), respect for all different knowledges in place, recognition of what needs to change/be transformed and sharing of experiences (i.e., spontaneous social interacting) for the integration of previous knowledge (experience) into 'new knowledge' (group commitment for action). Critical reflexive thinking in the context of the workshop intervention accepted the reality of the individuals' narratives and allowed the young people to re-evaluate their opinions, assumptions, and life expectations. It, thus, provided a path towards the recognition and acceptance for young people experiencing homelessness, from themselves and society. The significance of promoting trust for social engagement with services and within the community is apparent and reflects Islam et al.'s conceptualization of social capital [32]. In their concept of social capital, it is the need for mutually trusting networks, seen here as a consequence of the building of critical consciousness, which will provide a pathway for engagement with dental and health services, social services, and ultimately for social inclusion. In summary, trust building and social interacting appeared to transform relationships with services, strengthen social interacting, and enable critical reflexive thinking that, in turn, allowed for the subsequent production and acquisition of new knowledge and actions.

Theme 2: Constructing knowledge and developing skills

Giroux [33], in his exposition of Freire's critical pedagogy, makes a differentiation between gaining knowledge and the 'mastering of specific skills'. He states that Freire's approach is concerned with 'imaging literacy' and it is this 'mode of intervention [as] a way of learning [that can be used] as a basis for intervening in the world'. He goes on to describe that this process must 'afford [the individual] the opportunity to read, write and learn from a position of agency'. Doing so enables the attainment of information together with the creation and consolidation of new knowledge based upon 'the conditions of their current lives'. However, with the acquisition and consolidation of new knowledge we suggest that there was also skills development. Therefore, adopting Giroux's [33] position, a theme related to the acquisition and establishment of knowledge and skills development emerged from the data. For this second theme, the behavioral descriptors for knowledge were (i) 'information providing' and (ii) 'knowledge encoding'. These emerging themes were supported by Wolfe et al.'s [20] theory of health learning capacity, which has two main constructs that are associated with health cognitions and psychosocial skills (e.g., communication). The workshops allowed for knowledge skills development by enabling the participants to construct new knowledge through their reasoning (i.e., health cognitions) and verbal abilities (i.e., communications).

Theme 2 'constructing knowledge': using their life experiences, the young people reflected upon and encoded the content of the workshops. Verbally expressing their ideas on sensitive issues affecting them and listening to others, the young people increased critical thinking and improved their communication and conveyed their new knowledge to others. The young people, therefore, spoke of how the information was accessible and meaningful to them, encouraging new habits. The following comments are illustrative: 'I learnt about different foods' [workshop on health eating] (YP 4); 'I learnt about levels of sugar content in different drinks' (YP 10) [workshop on oral health]; 'I liked everything because I learnt a lot' (YP 1); 'It was really helpful' (YP 3); 'the best part of the workshop was to know how to overcome drug abuse and addiction' [workshop on substance misuse] (YP 1); and, 'I understand more about mental health' (YP 5) [workshop on mental health].

The inclusion of their own experiences, during constructing knowledge, permitted an encoding of the health information provided leading to an increased health awareness. The quote from a young man experiencing homelessness highlights this:

'I really enjoyed it because you talked about the use of cigarettes as well, the use of drugs, and that was really helpful for me to understand the effects that I will get after using drugs. So in that way it helped me to stay far from taking drugs. Really helpful to my health'. (YP 1)

Integrating the information into dynamic group activities thus afforded a platform for discussion ('I could talk about normal life, issues related to me'—YP 11) and enabled the construction of useful new personal knowledge, (as above), through the structuring of the information provided ('knowledge encoding'). Freeman [21] has postulated that it is within the context of people's social worlds that individuals are able to 'manipulate, encode and transform' health information into a useable form. The sharing of health information as part of knowledge encoding between young people and their service providers provided an opportunity for the converting of new information into an understandable and useable form. This was achieved by encouraging dialogue and the using of imaginative and diverse artistic learning activities to enable participants to express their feelings and opinions beyond the spoken word, therefore improving the psychosocial skill of communication. This was most apparent during the Resilience workshop that used a card game to build emotional strength. The young people had to choose and comment on quotes from famous people for transforming the thinking of their times:

"The session that I liked the most was the card games, yeah, that's true. There were quotes we had to choose, and I really liked the quote from Nelson Mandela saying about failures and stuff. The one on the importance of rising every time we fall. Yeah, it was really good to think about this". [the workshop on Resilience] (YP 6).

'I think the use of educational games was great. I particularly think the last session that we had on resilience was one of the best discussions I've had doing a group here. I mean the whole time I've been working here. Because it's very difficult to get young people to open up in that way and talk more widely about their bigger life goals and what they find scary. And I think the fact that they were happy to do so was a testament to the relationship that you've managed to build with them and also the resources available'. (SM 3)

Information providing and knowledge encoding, as descriptors for constructing knowledge, acted as precursors for 'developing skills' and behavior change. Skills development appeared to be associated with active learning, consensus building, and agreed action plans for future behavior change. Consensus building was an important dimension of knowing and it was used to combine group knowledge, for instance, for oral health-related behaviors.

"I was working with a young lad who came to a couple of the workshops, he had a workshop about dental health and a discussion about sugar and diet and stuff. And I know that he doesn't drink those energy drinks anymore, which is fantastic. Because he was drinking maybe one or two cans a day. And when you realize how much sugar was in them, because we had that visual exercise of how much sugar is in things, and I think that actually struck a chord with a few people, so I think that was really beneficial". (SM 5)

Therefore, the merging of old and new knowledge, within the group, supported new knowledge construction and its conversion into action plans for lifestyle change, as detailed in Table 3.

Table 3. Consensus building and joint action plans for oral health (OH) behavior change following OH workshop.

	Quotes Related with the Workshop on Oral Health
[1]	(I am) brushing my teeth differently (as a result of the workshop on how to brush teeth with fluoride toothpaste);
[2]	(I am) using mouthwash at different times [as a result of information about not using a mouthwash immediately after brushing teeth;
[3]	(I will) not use water when brushing my teeth as it'll wash away the concentrated fluoride in the remaining toothpaste' (as a result of the knowledge gained at the workshop);
[4]	'I now use a pea size of my toothpaste' (following the information given at the OH workshop when the facilitator asked a participant to show the right amount of toothpaste that should be used to brush the teeth and the amount showed was far away more than the recommended by NHS boards);
[5]	I am using a straw to drink any juice' (as result of the workshop on OH and diet that revealed the high amount of sugar present in the carbonated drinks consumed by the young people. The information caused a lot of surprise among the participants. The workshop provided advice on how to minimize the effects of these drinks with simple tips such as using a straw;

Theme 2 'knowledge conveying': the second behavior associated with the developing skills. Many of the young people suggested that they believed that they could tell, speak, or spread their new health knowledge among their friends and family:

"Basically, the main thing I've learned from the workshops, from being homeless and my journey is to respect and listen to other people because there are people who know more than you and you don't know everything. Take things that people say and take it on board, and everything's a learning curve, you learn things all the time... And I'd recommend that to anybody else who is homeless, just listen to other people, take on board what they've got to say, and accept the help that's around you like the group activity [the workshops]". (YP 3)

It may be suggested that a skill outcome of the workshop program was the strengthening of the young people's social interacting by equipping them with confidence to speak to others about health-related issues. This confirms the proposition that the workshop's pedagogical structure had provided the means by which young people could encode, transform, incorporate, and also disseminate new workshop information into a useful working knowledge language. For Wolf et al. [20], this would be evidence of improved health learning capacity: for Giroux's [33] it represents, 'a basis for intervening in the world':

"I think it's a very good thing [the workshops] because when you provide information about your own health, to people, it helps in their lives, and in that way you might help the same people who have got that information to tell other people... and these other people may someday come to get this information". (YP 6)

The participating staff members noted changes in the culture of the NGO following the program. They spoke of how the pedagogical workshops had provided them with new knowledge and increased their own awareness of the necessity of creating a supportive environment with and for young people:

"So I think the more we talk about people's health and how they can do things to help themselves, and more enabling stuff to give themselves the power into doing their own decision making in a positive way, then I think that should be strongly encouraged". (SM 1)

By joint working and the inclusion of people's rights and citizenship, as essential elements in health promotion interventions, they stated that the pedagogical workshop program had provided a strategy in the NGO to support young people who were experiencing homelessness. Moreover, there was a common understanding that all processes of change, especially those that are related with health improvement of people experiencing homelessness, were challenging for practitioners and service providers.

"I think sometimes health behaviors are some of the most difficult to change quite often I do come across young people who have got some pretty unhealthy habits in terms of smoking, eating, sleeping, that sort of thing but they do seem quite resistant to change". (SM 2)

4. Discussion

The aim of the work presented here was to use Freire's critical consciousness as an educative tool, to co-design, implement, and evaluate a series of pedagogical workshops to strengthen social interacting, critical consciousness, and to construct new knowledge, with, and for, homeless young people and their service providers. The findings showed the importance of incorporating this approach. The results intimated that shifts in self-regard and behavior of the young participants had occurred. Wider health topics and sensitive issues of their homelessness journeys were explored through their own lens in face of marginalization and exclusion. Regarding the delivery of the pedagogical workshop program, there was a positive and common feeling from the participants about key elements that were prioritized: the offer of a welcoming, safe, creative, and pleasant space to speak, share, and listen to other's narratives, and perceptions around each topic explored during the workshops. In this atmosphere, the participants were able to discuss issues that caused them concern and through the process of critical reflexion, collective construction of new knowledge and behaviors were achieved. The underpinning basis of the workshops was the adoption of a CRFA that connected oral health with other diverse topics. For example, the workshop on diet and nutrition was related to the consumption of sugars and hence oral health; the workshop on stigma brought up concerns about appearance of their teeth linked with social interaction and seeking employment opportunities, besides judgments made about their drug use and so reflected the concept of inclusion oral health. The importance of including the mental health workshop allowed dental anxiety, oral health-related quality of life and depression to be raised and explored by the participants. This was relevant, as previous research had shown that decayed and missing teeth were predictive of depression in homelessness [34]. Therefore, this workshop intervention was central to, among other aspects, the promotion of oral health, and health through increasing oral health literacy [20], to build trust among their peers and collective engaging with the service provider.

While this was realized using a process of mutual learning and the construction of new relationships, we suggest other factors were instrumental in establishing a safe and trustful place for spontaneous social interacting. A non-judgmental listening was crucial to involve vulnerable groups in discussions that affect their own health and wellbeing. We proposed that the safe place was created by 'locating [the participants] in the condition of their current lives' [33] together with increasing their awareness that they were not alone. The establishment of a place of safety to discuss sensitive issues, therefore, would appear to mimic a therapeutic space, which Bell et al. [35] consider to be of significance to 'maintain and promote health and wellbeing for different individuals and groups at different times'. It was within this therapeutic space that the assessment, re-assessment and reflection of past experiences, which had raised the levels of stigmatization and humiliation, were at last reconsidered, thereby reducing feelings of shame and inappropriateness [25,26]. We propose that critical consciousness as an educative tool conjured a therapeutic space for spontaneous social interacting—an 'empathetic encounter' to strengthen social engagement and consolidate new knowledge. In other words, the level of critical self-consciousness that was achieved by the young people had resulted in a better awareness of their relationship with their health and their wider attitudes as citizens.

In addition, some support for behavioral change was found. For instance, at the end of the workshop program, new health habits were noted in the participants through the post-questionnaire's evaluation and practitioners' feedback. Reports of speaking about, and sharing, difficult health and life experiences; critical reflexion on sensitive issues; working with others to form agreed action plans for health; together with the desire to act with peers and family to disseminate health messages, indicated to us that a behavioral shift had occurred. The young people became the 'problem-posers' or the questioners and as a consequence became involved in a dialogue about their oral health and wider health issues. The significance of this shift, while being related to their acquisition of new knowledge and improved self-regard, also aided young people to assist in changing the culture of the NGO. The main objective of the workshops was to offer to the participants a space for critical reflection on themes present in their lives in a welcoming, dynamic, and creative atmosphere that can encourage new actions and behaviors. The whole process follows the critical-reflexive line that was proposed by Freire, based on the integration of the previous knowledge of the young people with the appropriation of new and contextualized knowledge and practices.

Critical reflexion and confrontation of current life circumstances (in this case being young and homeless), as part of this critical consciousness proposed by Freire, allowed for participants to reflect upon their status, self-stigmatization, their responsibilities, and their roles in terms of social transformation. Young people and practitioners, thus, developed an increased understanding of the youth homelessness life context; how past health choices and experiences affects their current life and how this new knowledge acquisition strengthens future social change.

Limitations:

This work explored the use of a co-designed pedagogical workshop program to promote the acquisition of new knowledge and social interaction in a group of young people living in supported accommodation and attending activities that were provided by a NGO for homelessness.

A relatively small number of young homeless individuals took part and this calls into question the generalizability of the findings and conclusions to others experiencing social exclusion. However, while acknowledging the small sample size, this was a purposive and non-probability sample of a group of vulnerable homeless youth, who found it difficult to interact and engage with health and social care services and communities. They had, and were, experiencing social exclusion in diverse levels. The similarity of their comments and the merging themes suggested that saturation regarding their opinions and views of the workshops had been achieved and thus provided a form of validity to the findings. In addition, we were not able to comment on the longer-term behavior change at this stage of the research. Therefore, the findings of this qualitative evaluation provide a platform to allow future work on young vulnerable people, exploring co-designed interventions with this group to improve their engagement with services, health literacy, and enable social inclusion.

5. Conclusions

In conclusion, we propose that Freire's educational approach provides a useful framework to promote health and oral health with young people experiencing homelessness. It allowed the young people to be included in the co-design of the research intervention and enabled their active participation, building trust, and interaction with others within the NGO setting. In this process, opportunities to identify and to voice their health needs were explored, and their health learning capacity to make conscious, positive, and healthy choices was improved. Therefore, while accepting that there is a need for further research development in other NGO settings, this work suggests that the use of critical consciousness supports young socially excluded people's construction of new knowledge, health literacy, and strengthens their social interacting among their peers and engagement with services providers.

Other elements of this debate are related to the difficulties that are experienced with regard to behavior change among youths experiencing homelessness. We suggest that the development of agreed action plans during the workshops and subsequent noted behavior change were associated with the workshop program 'being located in the conditions of the current lives' of the service users and providers and the generation of a therapeutic space. It is expected that educational and research activities, such as the workshops, using Freire's theory, can contribute to listening to the voices of vulnerable and marginalized youths, encouraging them to adopt healthy life choices and also support them to achieve a critical consciousness and participatory citizenship.

Author Contributions: Conceptualization and principal investigator, A.R.; Workshop facilitators, A.R. and L.B.; Formal analysis, A.R. and R.F.; Funding acquisition, R.F.; Writing—original draft, A.R., L.B. and R.F.; Writing—review & editing, A.R., L.B. and R.F.

Funding: The Smile4life Programme was funded by the Scottish Government and National Health Service Boards, grant number: 121.80.4497. Support from NHS Education for Scotland; NHS Lothian; NHS Forth Valley; Cyrenians; CAIR Scotland and the Compass Project Team, Rock Trust and all participants.

Conflicts of Interest: The authors declare no conflict of interest.

References

1. BBC. Sofa Surfers: The Young Hidden Homeless. Available online: http://www.bbc.co.uk/news/uk42427398?intlink_from_url=http://www.bbc.co.uk/news/topics/c48yr9322xrt/homelessness&link_location=live-reporting-story (accessed on 22 December 2017).
2. Scottish Government. *Homelessness in Scotland: 2015–2016*; Scottish Government: Edinburgh, UK, 2016.
3. Scottish Government. Homelessness: Minister's Statement. Available online: https://beta.gov.scot/publications/ministerial-statement-on-homelessness-september-2017/ (accessed on 20 September 2017).
4. Scottish Government. A Nation with Ambition: The Government's Programme for Scotland 2017–2018. Available online: https://beta.gov.scot/publications/nation-ambition-governments-programme-scotland-2017-18/ (accessed on 20 September 2017).
5. Scottish Government. Policy: Homelessness. Available online: https://beta.gov.scot/policies/homelessness/ (accessed on 20 September 2017).
6. Scottish Government. Public Bodies (Joint Working) (Scotland) Act 2014. Available online: http://www.legislation.gov.uk/asp/2014/9/pdfs/asp_20140009_en.pdf (accessed on 10 May 2017).
7. Fitzpatrick, S.; Pawson, H.; Bramley, G.; Wilcox, S.; Watts, B. *The Homelessness Monitor: England 2017*; Crisis: London, UK, 2017.
8. Harleigh-Bell, N. *Youth Homelessness in Scotland 2015*; Homeless Action Scotland: Edinburgh, UK, 2016.
9. MacInnes, T.; Tinson, A.; Hughes, C.; Born, T.B.; Aldridge, H. Monitoring Poverty and Social Exclusion 2015. Available online: https://www.jrf.org.uk/mpse-2015 (accessed on 17 April 2017).
10. Homelessness Task Force. *Helping Homeless People: Legislative Proposals on Homelessness*; Scottish Executive: Edinburgh, UK, 2000.
11. Homelessness Task Force. *Helping Homeless People: An Action Plan for Prevention and Effective Response*; Scottish Executive: Edinburgh, UK, 2002.
12. Scottish Executive. Health and Homelessness Guidance. Available online: www.scotland.gov.uk/library3/health/hahg-00.asp (accessed on 17 April 2017).
13. Health Scotland. *Delivering Health Care to Homeless People: An Effectiveness Review (Research in Brief, 13)*; NHS Health Scotland: Edinburgh, UK, 2004.
14. Scottish Executive. *Health and Homelessness Standards*; Scottish Executive: Edinburgh, UK, 2005.
15. Sheiham, A.; Watt, R.G. The Common Risk Factor Approach: A rational basis for promoting oral health. *Community Dent. Oral Epidemiol.* **2000**, *28*, 399–406. [CrossRef] [PubMed]
16. Coles, E.; Themessl-Huber, M.; Freeman, R. Investigating community-based health and health promotion for homeless people: A mixed methods review. *Health Educ. Res.* **2012**, *27*, 624–644. [CrossRef] [PubMed]
17. Coles, E.; Freeman, R. Exploring the oral health experiences of homeless people: A deconstruction–reconstruction formulation. *Community Dent Oral Epidemiol.* **2016**, *44*, 53–63. [CrossRef] [PubMed]
18. Hudson, B.F.; Flemming, K.; Shulman, C.; Candy, B. Challenges to access and provision of palliative care for people who are homeless: A systematic review of qualitative research. *BMC Palliat. Care* **2016**, *15*, 96. [CrossRef] [PubMed]
19. Galea, N.K.; Kenyonb, S.; MacArthur, C.; Jolly, K.; Hope, L. Synthetic social support: Theorizing lay health worker interventions. *Soc. Sci. Med.* **2018**, *196*, 96–105. [CrossRef] [PubMed]
20. Wolf, M.S.; Wilson, E.A.; Rapp, D.N.; Waite, K.R.; Bocchini, M.V.; Davis, T.C.; Rudd, R.E. Literacy and learning in health care. *Pediatrics* **2009**, *124* (Suppl. 3), S275–S281. [CrossRef] [PubMed]

21. Freeman, R. Storytelling, sugar snacking, and toothbrushing rules: A proposed theoretical and developmental perspective on children's health and oral health literacy. *Int. J. Pediatr. Dent.* **2015**, *25*, 339–348. [CrossRef] [PubMed]
22. Freire, P. *Education for Critical Consciousness*; Bloomsbury Revelation Series: London, UK, 1974.
23. Freire, P. *Pedagogia do Oprimido*, 19th ed.; Paz e Terra: Rio de Janeiro, Brazil, 1991.
24. Candau, V.; Sacavino, S. *Educar em Direitos Humanos: Construir Democracia*; DP&A: Rio de Janeiro, Brazil, 2000.
25. Rodriguez, A. *Labyrinth of Trafficking: Lives, Practices and Interventions*; 7 Letras Publisher: Rio de Janeiro, Brazil, 2013.
26. Fernandes, F.L.; Rodriguez, A. The "lost generation" and the challenges in working with marginalized groups. Learnt lessons from Brazilian Favelas. *Radic. Community Work J.* 2015. Available online: http://www.rcwjournal.org/ojs/index.php/radcw/article/view/5 (accessed on 22 May 2018).
27. Labonte, R.; Laverack, G. Capacity building in health promotion, part 1: For whom? and for what purpose? *Crit. Public Health* **2001**, *11*, 111–127. [CrossRef]
28. Kidd, S.; Kral, M. Practicing participatory action research. *J. Couns. Psychol.* **2005**, *52*, 187–195. [CrossRef]
29. Rock Trust. Available online: http://www.rocktrust.org/about/ (accessed on 17 April 2016).
30. Marconi, M.A.; Lakatos, E.M. *Research Techniques: Planning and Execution of Research, Sampling and Research Techniques, Elaboration, Analysis and Interpretation of Data*; Atlas: São Paulo, Brazil, 2006. (In Portuguese)
31. Miles, M.B.; Huberman, I.; Saldana, J. *Qualitative Data Analysis: A Methods Sourcebook*, 3rd ed.; Sage Publications Ltd.: London, UK, 2014.
32. Islam, M.K.; Merlo, J.; Kawachi, I.; Lindström, M.; Gerdtham, U.G. Social capital and health: Does egalitarianism matter? A literature review. *Int. J. Equity Health* **2006**, *5*, 3. [CrossRef] [PubMed]
33. Giroux, H. Paulo Freire and the courage to be political. In *Reinventing Paulo Freire: A Pedagogy of Love*; Darder, A., Ed.; Routledge: New York, NY, USA, 2017.
34. Coles, E.; Chan, K.; Collins, J.; Humphris, G.M.; Richards, D.; Williams, B.; Freeman, R. Decayed and missing teeth and oral-health-related factors: Predicting depression in homeless people. *J. Psychosom. Res.* **2011**, *71*, 108–112. [CrossRef] [PubMed]
35. Bell, S.L.; Foley, R.; Houghton, F.; Maddrell, A.; Williams, A.M. From therapeutic landscapes to healthy spaces, places and practices: A scoping review. *Soc. Sci. Med.* **2018**, *196*, 123–130. [CrossRef] [PubMed]

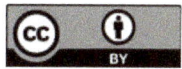

© 2019 by the authors. Licensee MDPI, Basel, Switzerland. This article is an open access article distributed under the terms and conditions of the Creative Commons Attribution (CC BY) license (http://creativecommons.org/licenses/by/4.0/).

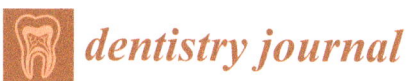

Article

Dental Attendance in Undocumented Immigrants before and after the Implementation of a Personal Assistance Program: A Cross-Sectional Observational Study

Martijn Lambert

Department of Community Dentistry and Oral Epidemiology, Special Needs in Oral Health, Ghent University, 9000 Ghent, Belgium; Martijn.Lambert@UGent.be; Tel.: +32-494-89-64-42

Received: 27 October 2018; Accepted: 11 December 2018; Published: 14 December 2018

Abstract: Undocumented immigrants are a high-risk social group with low access to care. The present study aims to increase awareness and dental attendance in this subgroup, assisted by community health workers (CHW). Starting from 2015, two trained dentists volunteered to perform free oral health examinations and further dental care referral in a welfare organisation in Ghent, Belgium. In 2016 and 2017, a two-day oral health training was added, enabling social workers to operate as community oral health workers and to provide personal oral health advice and assistance. Over the three years, an oral health examination was performed on 204 clients from 1 to 69 years old, with a mean age of 36.7 (SD = 15.9), showing high levels of untreated caries (71.6%; $n = 146$) and a Dutch Periodontal Screening Index (DPSI) score of 3 or 4 in 62.2% of the sample ($n = 97$). Regarding dental attendance, the total number of missed appointments decreased significantly, with 40.9% in 2015, 11.9% in 2016 and 8.0% in 2017 ($p < 0.001$). Undocumented immigrants can be integrated into professional oral health care. Personal assistance by community health workers might be an effective method, although this requires further investigation.

Keywords: undocumented immigrants; oral health care; community health workers

1. Introduction

Undocumented immigrants are a very vulnerable social subgroup, consisting of a considerable number of people trying to remain undiscovered by local authorities. In contrast to asylum seekers and recognised refugees, they do not have a residence permit to stay legally in the country. Their estimated number varies between 7% and 13% of the total number of immigrants with an official residence permit [1]. In Belgium, there were 1,214,605 legal immigrants on the 1 January 2014, which means that the number of undocumented immigrants probably lies between 85,000 and 160,000, corresponding to approximately 1% of the total Belgian population [2].

Although epidemiological data on the oral health of undocumented immigrants are scarce, some authors previously described the oral health and oral health needs of refugees in general [3–5]. According to these publications, oral diseases are highly prevalent in refugees and care provision is impeded by several barriers. It can be assumed that the oral health conditions of undocumented immigrants and their access to care are comparable or even worse, because they cannot register for an official health care insurance. However, according to the United Nations International Bill of Human Rights (1966), every individual has the right to "urgent medical care", including dental care, whether he or she has a residence status or not. Belgium ratified this universal human right and integrated it into its legislation in 1996.

In Belgium, the medical assistance provided to undocumented immigrants is financed by the federal government and organised at city level, and care can be both preventive and curative. To apply for it, people have to meet three criteria: they have been living for longer than three months in the country without permission to stay, they live in the city in which they apply for help, and they do not have a substantial income. In addition, a registered doctor or dentist needs to confirm the need for medical treatment.

Since the organisation of urgent medical care occurs at city level, there are local differences in care provision between different cities. In Ghent, Belgium, undocumented immigrants can obtain a "medical card", allowing them to receive medical treatments for a three month period, which can be repeated for as long as the three previously mentioned conditions are met. The medical card covers every treatment which is reimbursed by Belgian Social Security. Regarding dentistry, the medical card has two main shortcomings: it does not cover tooth extractions for people under the age of 53, nor provision of a removable denture for people under the age of 50.

The present survey originates from a purely voluntary-based project in "De Tinten", an organisation providing material and social assistance to illegal immigrants in Ghent, Belgium. In 2015, the organisation started to refer its clients to local dental clinics, driven by the high demand for dental care. However, the initial rate of missed appointments was so high (9 out of 22) that further collaboration between the organisation and the local dentists was put at stake.

In order to improve the system of referral and to increase dental attendance, the organisation set up a collaboration with researchers from Ghent university in 2016. To reduce barriers between both care providers and care demanders, the involvement of community health workers (CHW) was proposed. The involvement of CHWs in primary care showed to be an efficient way to guide underprivileged individuals towards preventive care and social services, reducing resource utilisation and community costs [6]. CHWs can also play an active role in oral health care. Benzian et al. composed a global competency matrix for oral health, involving many health professionals and groups in society, including CHWs [7]. Since oral health care provision in Belgium is almost exclusively founded upon the shoulders of the dentist, a CHW can be a valuable intermediary in oral health promotion and referral to oral health care. Greenberg et al. demonstrated the positive impact of dental case managers on Medicaid beneficiaries' (low-income individuals) use of dental services and the number of dentists participating in the Medicaid program [8].

The present survey aims to describe the preliminary results of referring undocumented immigrants to the dental practitioner, assisted by community health workers (CHW). Apart from reporting the oral health status of the participants, the main hypothesis is the following: Is the proportion of undocumented immigrants missing their appointment with external dentists the same before and after providing personal assistance?

2. Materials and Methods

The present cross-sectional study, which was based on annual convenience samples, describes the evolution in the proportion of missed dental appointments in undocumented immigrants in Ghent, Belgium, from February 2015 to December 2017. The study was carried out in "De Tinten", an organisation providing material and social assistance to undocumented immigrants in the city of Ghent.

Starting from February 2015, two trained dentists volunteered to perform free oral health examinations and dental interviews on a two-weekly base in a separated room in the organisation building. After oral consent, clients were interviewed on age, nationality and smoking habits. Nationalities were grouped according to the world health organization WHO (world health organization) regions. Individual oral health parameters included D_3MFT, which is the total number of decayed (at cavitation level), missing (due to caries) and filled teeth [9]. Based on the D_3MFT scores, a restorative index ($RI = (FT/(D_3 + FT)) \times 100$) and treatment index ($TI = (M + FT)/(D_3 + M + FT) \times 100$) were calculated in order to gain insights regarding the level of care. Severity of untreated dental caries was assessed using PUFA index, counting the number of teeth with visible pulp exposure, ulcerations, fistula and abscesses [10]. The plaque index of Sillness and Löe was used to measure the amount of dental plaque [11]. Periodontal health was assessed by using the Dutch Periodontal

Screening Index (DPSI) for participants older than 15 years old. This index describes the severity of periodontal disease (attachment loss around the teeth) and the need for further treatment on a scale from 0 to 4, after sounding the gums with a periodontal probe [12]. After the oral health examination, clients received a professional referral letter, as well as a dental goody bag, containing a toothbrush and toothpaste. Clients could apply for new toothpaste and a toothbrush every 8 weeks, even without oral health examination or referral. Before getting an appointment with an external dental clinic, all clients were required to obtain a "medical card" from the Ghent Social Welfare Organisation, confirming their undocumented status and allowing them to receive further medical care. Accordingly, only participants without a residence permit were included in the survey.

Starting from August 2016, the two-weekly oral health examinations remained unaltered, but the medical setting of the organisation changed, by training volunteers from the organisation to operate as community oral health workers. The training was held during a two-day program, and included provision of essential information on the normal development and anatomy of human dentition, oral diseases, preventive oral health, dental administration, motivational interviewing and case management. It was performed by two university researchers (one dentist and one psychologist), providing theoretical knowledge, clinical images, practical exercises and cases using an interactive PowerPoint presentation. In addition to the educational program, participants could consult and rehearse all information on a website (www.iedersmondgezond.be), which was specifically designed for the CHWs. As part of the website, a registration system was designed to follow up dental appointments. The information of this registration system was protected by a central log-in and password, and allowed the CHWs and the organisation to receive and send text messages when a client had a dental appointment in the upcoming 24 h.

The main task of the CHWs was to increase dental awareness and dental compliance among the undocumented immigrants, by completing all necessary administrative steps prior to the first dental visit, and by following up the further appointments. After the initial oral health examination, one of the CHWs called a local dentist to make an appointment in consultation with the client. When the appointment was made, it was registered in the digital registration system. Subsequently, the head of the organisation's medical service and the CHW considered whether the client needed personal assistance on the day of the appointment or not. The decision was made based on the linguistic capacities, personal competences and special needs of the individual client. In cases where doubt existed, or for first time visitors, personal assistance was always provided. When this personal assistance was required, the CHW received an expense allowance of €20 to cover transport and other direct costs.

At the end of the oral health examination, a referral letter was given to the client in case of need for further care. Clients were referred to the closest available dental office from their home address. When personal assistance was organised, a copy of the referral letter and the medical card of the client were given to the CHW in a closed envelope, in case the client lost or forgot it on the day of the appointment. If a second appointment was needed or the external dentist wanted to communicate directly with the organisation, the information was inserted in the closed envelope and returned to the organisation.

All external dentists were visited by the head of the medical service or contacted by phone before the first referral, in order to provide them with more information about the organisation and the involvement of CHWs. The dentists were informed and assured that the organisation would cover tooth extractions for people under the age of 53, which are not reimbursed by the government. Additionally, the dentists were allowed to apply for a "no show fee" in case of a missed appointment, which was also provided by the organisation.

The total number of appointments with external dentists was counted for 2015, 2016 and 2017. For each of these dental visits, the organisation registered whether the client was present or not. When an appointment was missed, the client was called by phone to ask for the reason for non-attendance. If the appointment was cancelled within the last 24 h, it was also considered as a missed appointment. Both the CHWs and the external dentists were asked to always contact the organisation in case of a missed appointment. When contacting the organisation, the external dentist could apply for a "no show fee" which was paid by the organisation. This fee ranged between €30 and €50, according to the dentist's standards.

Data analysis was carried in IBM SPSS Statistics V25.0 (SPSS Inc., Chicago, IL, USA). After explorative data analyses, differences in proportions were examined using crosstabs and Chi-square statistical tests. Alpha was set at 0.05.

The study was approved by the Ethics Committee of the University Hospital Ghent (B670201526486). All subjects gave their informed consent for inclusion before they participated in the study. They received a referral letter and were supported to visit a dentist when further care was needed. Clinical data were stored in a database specifically designed for the survey, using VTiger CRM system 7.1.0RC. The data, including personal data, were protected by an external hosting company and could not be consulted or modified by a third party. Before data analysis, all records were encrypted to ensure anonymity.

3. Results

Over the three years, an oral health examination was performed on 204 clients from 1 to 69 years old, with a mean age of 36.3 (Standard Deviation (SD) = 15.9). Baseline characteristics are indicated in Table 1. Untreated tooth caries were visible in 71.6% ($N = 146$) of the participants ($D_3 > 0$). From those with tooth decay, 46.7% had at least one tooth with visible pulpal exposure. The level of care was low, with an average restorative index of 30.3% (SD = 36.9) and a treatment index of 51.5% (SD = 37.9). Periodontal health was poor, with 62.2% ($N = 97$) of the clients having a DPSI score of 3 or 4.

Table 1. Characteristics of the examined sample.

Total Sample		$N = 204$	
	Mean	SD	Missing
Age	36.3	15.9	$N = 35$
Years in Belgium	4.6	4.7	$N = 0$
Plaque Index	1.4	0.8	$N = 18$
DPSI *	2.6	1.1	$N = 16$
D_3MFT	9.4	8.4	$N = 0$
PUFA	1.6	3.0	$N = 0$
Restorative Index	30.3	36.9	$N = 39$
Treatment Index	51.5	37.9	$N = 28$
Number of teeth with active caries per person	3.4	3.9	$N = 0$
Number of teeth with visual pulp exposure per person	1.3	2.5	$N = 0$
	Valid %	N	Missing
Origin (WHO region)	-	-	$N = 11$
African Region	11.9	23	-
Region of the Americas	1.0	2	-
South-East Asia Region	0.5	1	-
European Region	67.4	130	-
Eastern Mediterranean Region	37	19.2	-
Western Pacific Region	0.0	0	-
Smoker **	-	-	$N = 20$
Yes	46.2	60	-
No	52.3	68	-
Former smoker	1.5	2	-
Gender	-	-	$N = 10$
Male	44.3	108	-
Female	55.7	86	-
Active tooth decay	-	-	$N = 0$
Present	71.6	146	-
Not Present	28.4	58	-
Visible pulp Exposure	-	-	$N = 0$
Present	35.8	73	-
Not Present	64.2	131	-

* From those > 15 years old ($N = 143$); ** From those > 12 years old ($N = 150$).

Regarding dental attendance during the survey period, Figure 1 and Table 2 illustrate the number of external appointments provided to the target population for 2015, 2016 and 2017. The avoidable missed appointments without acceptable reason are indicated in red (Figure 1), the others in green. The orange bar indicates the number of missed appointments with legitimate reasons.

According to Table 2, the organisation registered 176 appointments with 16 different external dental practices in 2017, of which 89 were first dental visits. Physical assistance was provided for 87 appointments. Over the three years, the total number of missed appointments decreased significantly, with 40.9% in 2015, 11.9% in 2016 and 8.0% in 2017 ($p < 0.001$). The percentage of avoidable missed appointments dropped to 3.4%.

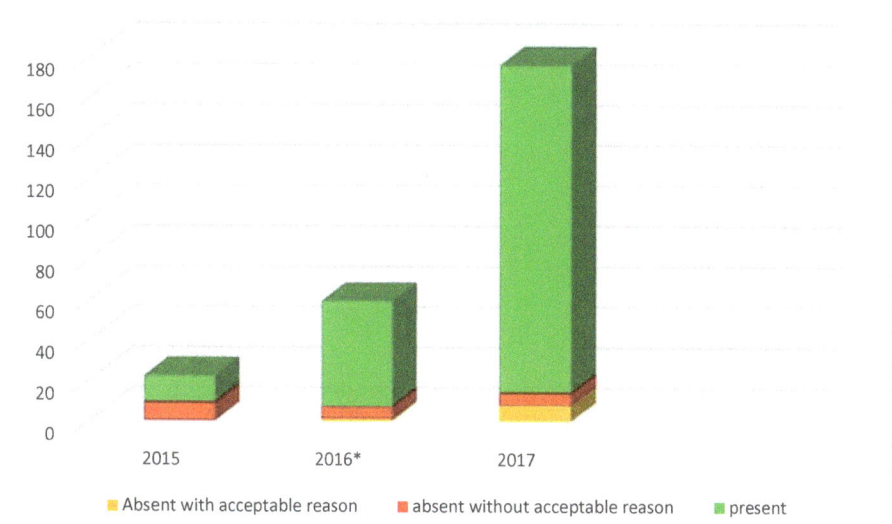

Figure 1. The number of appointments made with external dental practitioners and the proportion of missed appointments (y-axis) over the three study years (x-axis). *In August 2016, the personal assistance program was implemented.

Table 2. Total number of appointments for 2015, 2016 and 2017, and the proportion and explanation of missed appointments.

Appointments	2015	2016	2017
Total number of appointments	22 (100%)	59 (100%)	176 (100%)
Client present	13 (59.1%) *	52 (88.1%) *	162 (92.0%) *
Client absent	9 (40.9%)	7 (11.9%)	14 (8.0%)
Client absent without acceptable reason	9 (40.9%)	6 (10.2%)	6 (3.4%)
Client absent with acceptable reason	0 (0.0%)	1 (1.7%)	8 (4.5%)
Cancellation >24 h before appointment	-	-	4 (2.3%)
Unforeseen circumstances (arrestation, hospitalisation)	-	1 (1.7%)	2 (1.1%)
Error made by organisation or dentist			2 (1.1%)

* $p < 0.001$ according to chi-square test.

4. Discussion

The cross-sectional survey presented annual convenience samples within a Belgian organisation for undocumented immigrants. The participants were mainly young, with a mean age of 36.3. Their initial oral health care needs are considerable, as seen in Table 1. The presence of tooth decay was very high, with untreated decay at cavitation level ($D_3 > 0$) being present in 71.6% of the records, of which half had visible pulp exposure. Periodontal health was very poor, especially taking into account the mean age of 36.7, with 62.2% ($N = 97$) of participants having a DPSI score of 3 or 4. The bad periodontal condition can be partially explained by the high number of smokers (46.2%). Although the present oral health outcomes are alarming, they should be interpreted with caution. The present survey used a convenience sample, which means that the observed findings cannot be generalized for all undocumented immigrants, not even within the organisation. It can be assumed that people with high dental needs will be more likely to accept the offer of a dental screening and further referral, leading to selection bias and partially declaring the high level of tooth decay and periodontal disease in the initial examinations. No information was available from non-responders.

In contrast to the high dental need, the initial care level was almost negligible before the intervention. Although the present survey cannot draw conclusions on the causes of care avoidance, several determinants might play a role. First of all, the illegal character of the participants' residence forces them to hide from most official institutions. To get medical care, they need to present themselves to the local authorities. Although no one can ever be arrested while seeking help in one of these centres, officially registering for (oral) health care can still be a barrier. Furthermore, living in precarious conditions might also have an influence. As one of the most underprivileged groups in society, people without a residence permit suffer from the same social determinants which are mainly associated with deprived oral health: material deprivation, educational attainment, origin, professional status, and the lack of a social network. These factors are largely described in international literature as predictors of adverse oral health outcomes [13,14]. Since the average time of living in Belgium was almost five years in the presented sample, it is very likely that the adverse living conditions have played an important role in the oral health outcomes.

To support the target population, the intervention aimed to enable social workers, having a close relationship with the undocumented immigrants, to be involved in oral health care as community health workers. Since community health workers are people known by the target population, providing food and other assistance, they might have more authority and get more trust than an external caregiver. Acting as a contact person between care demander and care provider, the community oral health workers also consider the barriers perceived by the local dentists. Emphasis was put on adequate information and translation, and on the reduction of administrative burden and the number of missed appointments. Bedos et al. previously reported that frustrations expressed by dentists mainly concern missed appointments, difficulties in performing non-covered treatments and low government fees [15]. In our intervention, every dentist was called or visited personally by the head of the medical service of the organisation. During this conversation, the dentist could express his personal expectations and concerns, which were taken into account by the organisation and the CHWs. For example, when a dentist indicated not to speak French or English, the organisation only sent clients who were able to speak Dutch, or who were accompanied by a Dutch-speaking translator. The personal approach and mutual empathy resulted in a considerable network of 16 dentists accepting the undocumented immigrants in their dental practice. This can be considered a success, since the number of general dentists in Flanders is decreasing and dental practitioners are ageing. In 2017, the estimated number of qualified dentists was 1 per 1147 residents in Belgium and 1 per 1182 in Flanders (http://www.dekamer.be/QRVA/pdf/54/54K0138.pdf, p261). Furthermore, Belgium has until present no experience with dental hygienists as part of the professional dental team. When the number of dentists decreases, it can be assumed that the "law of demand and supply" will not be beneficial to vulnerable subgroups in society, such as undocumented immigrants.

Aiming to cope with the high unmet oral health needs and various user-side and supplier-side barriers, one of the major strengths of the present intervention was the creation of a safe and reliable partnership between the organisation and both the target population and the local dentists. Concerning the undocumented immigrants, the key elements of the intervention were outreach work, personal assistance and the involvement of existing networks. Indeed, oral health behaviour and oral health in general are largely affected by social networks and social support, defined as people's "social capital" [16].

Although the first results of the involvement of CHWs suggest a reduction in barriers towards dental care provision in both undocumented immigrants and local dentists, the effects might not be automatically applicable. Care provision strongly depends on national policy and health care budgets. According to a report of Cuadra, access to health care for undocumented immigrants varies between European countries [17]. Some countries, such as Belgium, only provide the minimum as set out by the UN Human Rights and specified by article 13.2 of the "Council of Europe Resolution 1509 (2006) on Human Rights of Irregular Migrants", whereas other countries provide more or sometimes less than this minimum access to care.

Even in Belgium, the results of the intervention might differ between cities. Since medical care for undocumented immigrants is organised at city level, inequalities in care provision between cities are probable, although this requires further investigation. The medical card in Ghent is an accessible instrument to help undocumented immigrants, but it does not exist in other cities such as Antwerp or Brussels, where decisions on reimbursement depend on each individual case. It is recommendable to obtain clear and equal legislation on a national scale, to avoid inequity and possible delocalisation of undocumented immigrants from one city to another. Medical care should not be determined by place of residence.

Although the medical card in Ghent might be an easy instrument to get access to dental care, the lack of coverage for tooth extractions for people under the age of 53 is a limitation, leading to high out-of-pocket costs. For 2017, the local organisation "De Tinten" spent €2311 of its own budget on no-show fees and uncovered basic treatment costs (excluding prosthodontic treatments), and paid €1616 for personal assistance by CHWs, yielding an average cost of €22.31 per appointment. Without external charity funding, this intervention could be compromised.

In order to reduce curative treatment costs in the future, the intervention did not focus exclusively on guiding clients to the dental office, but CHWs were trained during the educational program to pay attention to preventive oral health care and oral health behaviour. Furthermore, free dental goody bags were provided on a regular basis (every eight weeks). Budgets for preventive materials amounted to €2130 in 2017 and were also paid for by charity funding. It needs further research to investigate if this intervention can lead to a reduction of the overall costs in the long term due to improved oral health outcomes.

The present survey has some important limitations to report. Regarding the positive dental attendance rates in 2017, these results should be interpreted with caution. Increased dental attendance might not automatically imply increased dental awareness, better oral health behaviours or improved oral health outcomes, especially in the long term. Furthermore, the use of the words "urgent medical care" in legislation might also impede the mindset shift from curative care and falling from one oral health problem into the other, towards more cost saving preventive care. Although the law states that "urgent medical care" can be both curative and preventive, policy makers and stakeholders tend to consider preventive check-ups, supragingival scaling and small fillings as "non-urgent". Even some dental practitioners feel reluctant to sign the required form to confirm that their treatment was urgent. The author suggests that "necessary medical care" would be a better wording than "urgent medical care", avoiding semantic discussions and professional neglect of painless lesions.

Secondly, the survey could not link the external appointments to the original and individual characteristics of the clients, due to technical limitations. This makes it impossible to know if there were specific personal or oral health determinants, leading to more missed appointments. Furthermore, the present survey cannot provide information on responders and non-responders within the target population. The invitation to participate in the survey aimed to be as accessible as possible to undocumented immigrants. In order not to frighten them, it was impossible to make official lists and numbers of all undocumented immigrants who could possibly be involved. Furthermore, the recruitment process was carried out over several weeks during food distribution, making it impossible to count the total number of unique clients in this setting. Nevertheless, it is possible that the invitation attracted the most motivated clients, leading to higher rates of dental attendance.

As a final limitation, the present study is not a randomised controlled trial, exploring differences in outcomes between an intervention and control group over the same study period. Comparing different convenience samples before and after a program without the use of a proper control group inevitably leads to reporting bias. The absence of a control group was due to ethical reasons. The initial rates of missed appointments in 2015 (40.9%) negatively affected the reputation of undocumented immigrants among local dentists. Since there is no dental public health system in Belgium, all residents, legal and illegal, entirely depend on care from private dentists. If a control group was used, in which the number of missed appointments would remain high during some more years, it would be possible that local dentists would turn against all undocumented immigrants because of those in the control group. In real life circumstances, dealing with extremely vulnerable human beings, this was a risk nobody wanted to take.

Despite the clear scientific shortcomings of the survey, it is difficult to assume that the dramatic decrease in missed appointments over the two years would be due to factors other than the reported intervention. Even if this was due to other factors, the present survey shows that undocumented immigrants can be integrated into regular dental care and that high levels of dental attendance can be achieved in this population.

5. Conclusions

The present sample of undocumented immigrants shows very poor oral health, both in terms of tooth decay and periodontal disease. However, the decreasing proportions of missed appointments indicate that undocumented immigrants can be integrated into professional oral health care. Personal assistance by community health workers might be an effective method, although this requires further investigation.

Funding: This research received no external funding.

Acknowledgments: The author wants to acknowledge the indispensable support, dedication and innovative long term vision on oral and general health which is demonstrated by the medical and social service of "De Tinten", by providing high-quality assistance to undocumented immigrants on a voluntary basis.

Conflicts of Interest: The author declares no conflict of interest.

References

1. Triandafyllidou, A. Clandestino Project—Final Report. Available online: http://clandestino.eliamep.gr/wp-content/uploads/2010/03/clandestino-final-report_-november-20091.pdf (accessed on 13 December 2018).
2. Baeyens, P.; Beys, M.; Bourguignon, M.; Büchler, A.; De Smet, F.; Dewulf, K.; Dutilleux, A.; Gaspart, G.; Lejeune, J.; Swankaert, J.; et al. Migration en droits et en chiffres 2015-Migratie in cijfers en in rechten 2015. Available online: https://www.myria.be/files/Migration-rapport_2015-LR.pdf (accessed on 13 December 2018).
3. Keboa, M.T.; Hiles, N.; Macdonald, M.E. The oral health of refugees and asylum seekers: A scoping review. *Glob. Health* **2016**, *12*, 59. [CrossRef]
4. Van Berlaer, G.; Bohle Carbonell, F.; Manantsoa, S.; De Béthune, X.; Buyl, R.; Debacker, M.; Hubloue, I. A refugee camp in the centre of Europe: Clinical characteristics of asylum seekers arriving in Brussels. *BMJ Open* **2016**, *6*, e013963. [CrossRef]
5. Riggs, E.; Rajan, S.; Casey, S.; Kilpatrick, N. Refugee child oral health. *Oral Dis.* **2017**, *23*, 292–299. [CrossRef] [PubMed]
6. Johnson, D.; Saavedra, P.; Sun, E.; Stageman, A.; Grovet, D.; Alfero, C.; Maynes, C.; Skipper, B.; Powell, W.; Kaufman, A. Community Health Workers and Medicaid Managed Care in New Mexico. *J Community Health* **2012**, *37*, 563–571. [CrossRef] [PubMed]
7. Benzian, H.; Greenspan, J.S.; Barrow, J.; Hutter, J.W.; Loomer, P.M.; Stauf, N.; Perry, D.A. A competency matrix for global oral health. *J. Dent. Educ.* **2015**, *79*, 353–361. [PubMed]

8. Greenberg, B.J.S.; Kumar, J.V.; Stevenson, H. Dental case management—Increasing access to oral health care for families and children with low incomes. *JAMA* **2008**, *139*, 1114–1121.
9. Klein, H.T.; Palmer, C.E.; Knutson, J.W. Studies on dental caries I dental status and dental needs of alimentary school children. *Public Health Rep.* **1938**, *53*, 751–765. [CrossRef]
10. Monse, B.; Heinrich-Weltzien, R.; Benzian, H.; Holmgren, C.; van Palenstein Helderman, W. PUFA—An index of clinical consequences of untreated dental caries. *Community Dent. Oral Epidemiol.* **2010**, *38*, 77–82. [CrossRef] [PubMed]
11. Silness, J.; Löe, H. Correlation between oral hygiene and periodontal condition. *Acta Odontol. Scand.* **1964**, *22*, 121–135. [CrossRef] [PubMed]
12. Van der Velden, U. The Dutch periodontal screening index validation and its application in The Netherlands. *J. Clin. Periodontol.* **2009**, *36*, 1018–1024. [CrossRef] [PubMed]
13. Sanders, A.E.; Slade, G.D.; Turrell, G.; Spencer, A.J.; Marcenes, W. The shape of the socio-economic-oral health gradient: Implications for theoretical explanations. *Community Dent. Oral Epidemiol.* **2006**, *34*, 310–319. [CrossRef] [PubMed]
14. Schwendicke, F.; Dörfer, C.E.; Schlattmann, P.; Page, L.F.; Thomson, W.M.; Paris, S. Socio-economic inequality and caries: A systematic review and meta-analysis. *J. Dent. Res.* **2015**, *94*, 10–18. [CrossRef] [PubMed]
15. Bedos, C.; Loignon, C.; Landry, A.; Richard, L.; Allison, P.J. Providing care to people on social assistance: How dentists in Montreal, Canada, respond to organisational, biomedical, and financial challenges. *BMC Health Serv. Res.* **2014**, *14*, 472. [CrossRef] [PubMed]
16. Rouxel, P.L.; Heilmann, A.; Aida, J.; Tsakos, G.; Watt, R.G. Social capital: Theory, evidence, and implications for oral health. *Community Dent. Oral Epidemiol.* **2015**, *43*, 97–105. [CrossRef] [PubMed]
17. Cuadra, C.B. Right of access to health care for undocumented migrants in EU: A comparative study of national policies. *Eur. J. Public Health* **2012**, *22*, 267–271. [CrossRef] [PubMed]

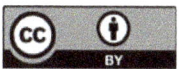 © 2018 by the author. Licensee MDPI, Basel, Switzerland. This article is an open access article distributed under the terms and conditions of the Creative Commons Attribution (CC BY) license (http://creativecommons.org/licenses/by/4.0/).

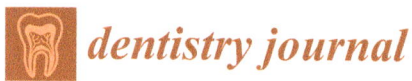

Article

Evaluating an Oral Health Education Intervention in Chinese Undocumented Migrant Mothers of Infants in Northern Ireland

Siyang Yuan

Dental Health Services Research Unit, School of Dentistry, University of Dundee, Park Place, Dundee DD1 4HN, UK; s.z.yuan@dundee.ac.uk

Received: 19 November 2018; Accepted: 14 January 2019; Published: 19 January 2019

Abstract: Background: Poor oral health remains a significant dental public health challenge for ethnic minority and immigrant groups living in the UK. This study aimed to evaluate a culturally appropriate community-based home visiting oral health education intervention for Chinese, undocumented migrant mothers to promote their infants' oral health, by focusing on their oral health related knowledge, attitudes, and behaviors. Methods: A convenience sample of 36 Chinese mothers with babies aged less than eight weeks were recruited in South-East region of Belfast. The local Chinese community was consulted to assist with the development of the intervention. The oral health education intervention was provided to 19 intervention group mothers through home visits and telephone calls during mothers' first postpartum year. They were also provided with unlimited social support during the intervention period. Mothers' oral health related knowledge, attitudes, and behaviors regarding baby toothbrushing and sugar snacking were measured at eight weeks, six months, and 12 months. Results: A higher proportion of Chinese intervention group mothers had improved knowledge about baby toothbrushing at 12 months compared with control group mothers (χ^2 = 14.12: p = 0.004). Significantly, more intervention group mothers' oral health related attitudes were enhanced regarding baby toothbrushing and sugar snacking compared with control group mothers. Conclusion: This community-based oral health education intervention has shown effects in mothers' self-reported knowledge, attitudes, and behaviors in the intervention group when the community based and culturally appropriate home-visiting program improved the mothers' oral health related knowledge, attitudes, and behaviors.

Keywords: undocumented migrant; baby oral health; oral health education; parental knowledge; attitudes and behaviors

---

1. Introduction

Untreated dental caries has been shown to be the greatest disease burden in the world, with untreated caries of deciduous teeth ranked as the 10th greatest global disease burden [1]. As a consequence, children suffer poor oral health and poor quality of life, especially for those from socially disadvantaged backgrounds [2].

The association between socioeconomic status (SES) and health outcomes has been well established and it further affected by such factors as ethnicity [3,4]. For decades, research on ethnic disparities in health has provided evidence that health inequalities may decrease or even disappear if SES inequalities were eliminated [5]. However, in recent years, the focus on racial/ethnic health inequalities has shifted from "race or class" to the intersectionality between race/ethnicity and class [6]. For example, findings from a longitudinal study of a birth cohort showed that health gains from improved family economic resources were smaller for Black than for White young people [7]. Similarly the effects of parental education on families' functioning to escape poverty was larger for

White compared to Black [8]. Based on the 'Diminished Return theory for Minorities', race/ethnicity and SES are two different and interrelating factors of social position that may explain the role of racial/ethnic upon health inequities [6,9].

During the migration process, immigrant families face multiple disadvantages when adapting to the host society in terms of lifestyle and cultural norms. These disadvantages include financial hardship for settlement, language difficulty, little knowledge of available social, and healthcare resources and psychosocial stress caused by their unsettled immigration status. With regard to oral health, migrant children have been shown to have poorer oral health outcomes compared with children in the host country [10]. It has been suggested that this may be due to the fact that migrant childhood is exposed to multiple disadvantages during the migration process, which had adverse consequences for growth and health. As possible consequences of these socioeconomic and cultural disadvantages, children from newly arrived immigrant families are more likely to suffer the poorest oral health. A recent Australian study showed that length of time as a resident in the host country was an independent predictor for the preschool children's obvious caries experience [11].

An additional factor in a child's obvious decay experience is the association between maternal oral health related knowledge, beliefs and practices, and child oral health [12–15]. Furthermore, mother's cariogenic bacteria can be transmitted to the child, which has been shown in the association of maternal and child's levels of Streptococcus mutans (MS) [16]. Other studies have reported an association between children's caries experience and their mothers' poor oral health status [13,16]. More significantly, mothers who do not appreciate the importance of child oral health are less likely to brush their children's teeth with fluoride toothpaste [16]. It is therefore of importance to address these factors when designing a community-based oral health promotion intervention to improve parents' oral health related knowledge, attitudes, and behaviors regarding child oral health.

Unfortunately, little research investigating, specifically, Chinese migrant parents' oral health related knowledge, beliefs, and practices are available. Wong et al. explored Chinese parents' perceptions regarding oral hygiene and access to dental care. They found that parents had proper knowledge about the best feeding practice and had fatalistic attitudes toward child tooth decay [17]. The lack of oral health related knowledge and positive attitudes created barriers for Chinese parents when they sought preventive dental care for their young children. Wong et al.'s findings further underscore the need of an oral health promotion intervention that is culturally appropriate for Chinese migrant parents [17].

Community-based interventions, such as home visiting programs, have been demonstrated to be effective in raising parental awareness of, and assisting them to, adopt healthy lifestyle behaviors that are beneficial to children's health needs [18–20]. Using a one-to-one health educational approach, community health workers who are from similar ethnic and social backgrounds will be more likely to understand the psycho-social difficulties, concerns, and health needs of newly arrived immigrant families. This, as proposed, will build up trusting relationships between parents and oral health professionals and will enable the delivery of oral health messages.

The aim of this study therefore was to examine the effect of a community-based, home visiting oral health education intervention delivered in a culturally appropriate approach for Chinese newly arrived undocumented migrant mothers. It focused on promoting mothers' oral health related knowledge, their intentions to brush their babies' teeth with fluoride toothpaste and to control baby sugar snacking, their oral health related behaviors as well as their own oral health in terms of obvious decayed experience.

2. Materials and Methods

2.1. Study Design and Setting

The study design was a quasi-experimental study with no randomization of the participating Chinese newly arrived undocumented migrant mothers. Undocumented migrants are people who are living without a valid residence permit authorizing them to permanently stay in the country in which they are currently residing [21]. The study setting was in the South and West regions of Belfast in the UK. In Northern Ireland (NI), Chinese migrant group constitutes the largest ethnic group with an approximately size of population of 8000 [22]. The majority of the Chinese population originate from Hong Kong and have been residents in NI since the 1960s. However in recent years, Chinese people from Northern region of Fu Jian province of Southern China, one of the most deprived areas in China, have migrated to NI. Most of the Fu Jian men work in catering services for long hours with low pay. The Fu Jian undocumented migrant mothers are unable to speak much English and remain at home most of the time.

In terms of the dental health care system in Northern Ireland, people have to pay for their dental treatments unless they are entitled to free National Health Service (NHS) dental treatments [23]. For example, it is free for children under 18 and pregnant women as well as women with babies aged up to 12 months to receive dental examinations and treatments in NHS dental care services.

2.2. Sample

A sample size of 17 Chinese migrant mothers in the intervention group, and 17 in the control group, was calculated to have 80% power to detect a difference in the caries incidence of 0.56 between the intervention and control group mothers' D_3MFT assuming that the common standard deviation is 0.55 using a two-group t-test with 0.05 two-sided significance level.

On statistical advice, the control group mothers were recruited six months before the recruitment of intervention group mothers. This was to reduce the possibility of contamination from this oral health education intervention. The intervention group mothers were selected to match the demographic profile (i.e., mother's age, educational attainment, level of relative deprivation, etc.) of the control group mothers. Both intervention and control group mothers have been settled in the UK for no longer than three years. All participants were undocumented migrants. A "snowball sampling" technique was used in order to recruit this 'hard to reach' group of newly arrived undocumented migrant mothers [24]. This strategy relied on the initial participating mothers to provide access to other members of their group or community by word of mouth.

2.3. Intervention Program

The intervention aimed to promote Chinese newly arrived, undocumented migrant mothers' oral health related knowledge, their intentions to brush baby's teeth using fluoride toothpaste and to control baby sugar consumption, and their oral health related behaviors in the first 12 months of the baby's life. Therefore, prior to the development of the program, the Chinese Welfare Association and community leaders were contacted. The nature of the program was explained and advice requested. Using the information received from talking with Chinese migrant mothers with toddlers born in Belfast and understanding their health and social needs, the program was formulated.

The community-based oral health education intervention was delivered by a Chinese community health worker (SY) in a culturally appropriate way through home visiting and telephone contact at five different time points over the intervention period (Table 1). During the home visits, SY provided information about oral health focusing on promoting healthy feeding (including introducing suitable foods and drinks for the benefits of baby's teeth), baby teething, and benefit of twice daily toothbrushing using fluoride toothpaste as well as regular dental attendance for both mothers and babies. She also demonstrated the correct toothbrushing techniques to the mothers in the intervention group and encouraged them to use the teething and oral hygiene resources as well as a trainer cup. These were provided during the intervention. In addition, the trust between the Chinese health worker and mothers was built throughout the intervention period and social support provided, based on mothers' needs such as referring them to the local social services and health and/or oral health services.

Table 1. The procedures of the intervention program [25].

Infants' Age	Intervention Tasks	Support Materials Provided
8 weeks	The community health worker is to: • provide breastfeeding advice; • provide weaning information; • give oral health advice about baby teething, mother's oral hygiene and regular dental attendance; • encourage mothers to see a dentist and brush their teeth at least twice a day.	1. UNICEF Breastfeeding information leaflet; 2. Weaning information leaflet; 3. Baby teething ring; 4. Mother's toothbrush and fluoride toothpaste
4 months	A telephone call was made to reinforce the information given at 8 weeks	
6 months	The community health worker is to: • emphasize the need to start to brush baby's teeth with a smear of fluoride toothpaste as soon as first teeth erupt; • demonstration of baby toothbrushing with emphasis on the smear size of fluoride toothpaste on baby; • emphasize the benefits of introducing a feeding cup from 6 months onwards rather than a bottle; • give advice on suitable foods and drinks for the benefits of baby's teeth.	1. Baby trainer cup; 2. Oral health pack containing baby toothbrush and fluoride toothpaste; 3. Mother's toothbrush and fluoride toothpaste.
9 months	A telephone call was made to reinforce the information given at 6 months	
12 months	The community health worker thanked mothers for their participation.	1. Baby feeding cup; 2. Toothbrushes and fluoride toothpaste for mothers and child

2.4. Data Collection

2.4.1. Questionnaire

The questionnaire was developed in several parts, which included demographic information, assessments of the mother's oral health related knowledge, attitudes, and behaviors. Mothers' demographics included information such as their age, marital status and postal codes of their residential areas. The post code would enable an assessment of social deprivation to be made using the Noble Index of Deprivation [22]. The Noble Index of Deprivation is a multiple deprivation measure that includes information from the seven domains of: Income, employment, health and disability, education skills and training, proximity to services, living environment, and crime and disorder.

The attitudinal items were assessed on a five-point Likert scale ranging from "strongly disagree" (scoring 1) through "neither agree nor disagree" (scoring 3) to "strongly agree" (scoring 5). These questions were derived from previous studies and had a good reliability and validity [26]. The questionnaire contained one oral health related knowledge question with a single choice answer at the baseline assessment regarding the age of babies that mothers think they should start brushing baby's teeth. A section was included for the six-month and 12-month questionnaire assessments to evaluate mothers' knowledge and behaviors with regard to baby toothbrushing using fluoride toothpaste. If the mother answered 'Yes', then she would be asked to complete this section about baby toothbrushing;

otherwise she would be advised to go to the next section of the questionnaire. Questions regarding mothers' own oral health related behaviors such as toothbrushing behavior and dental attendance were included in the questionnaires using single choice answers such as "how many times do you brush your teeth during the day?" and "what is your usual reason for going to see a dentist?".

2.4.2. Assessment of Mothers' Dental Health Status

Prior to the evaluation, an independent and calibrated dental examiner (AS) who was blind with regard to the aim of the study was invited to examine all the participants' teeth. After training and calibration, AS's intra-examiner reliability was 0.94 (Kappa value).

Mother's dental health status was assessed using obvious decay experience (D_3MFT). The protocol used recognizes decay, which extends into the dentine on the basis of a clinical examination conducted without the use of probes [27]. Dental caries were diagnosed at the decay into dentine (D_3) threshold using a visual method (including visual dentine caries) without radiography, fiber-optic transillumination, or compressed air. The mothers' teeth were inspected under standardized illumination. The calibrated dental examiner (AS) used a flexi-lum light and mouth mirror. All necessary steps were taken to prevent cross-infection. For example, disposable gloves and disposable mirrors were used and collected in medical waste bags and were disposed of in hospital.

2.4.3. Outcome Measures

The primary outcome measures were mothers' oral health related knowledge, attitudes and behaviors with regard to baby toothbrushing, sugar consumption and baby tooth decay as well as maternal dental health behaviors, measured at eight weeks, six months, and 12 months. The secondary outcome measure was mothers' obvious decay experience examined at eight weeks, six months, and 12 months.

2.5. Ethical Considerations

Ethical approval was granted from the Office for Research Ethics Committees Northern Ireland (Ref: 05/NIR02/64). All subjects gave their informed consent for inclusion before they participated in the study.

2.6. Statistical Analysis

Data from questionnaires were entered into SPSS 12.0.1. Frequencies were computed to describe the demographic profile of mothers of babies. Mother's attitudinal questions regarding their intentions to brush baby's teeth using fluoride toothpaste and to control baby sugar consumption were summed according to the Likert scales developed from factor analyses from the previous study [26]. Chi-squared analysis and Fisher's exact test was used to compare mothers' oral health related knowledge and self-reported behaviors between intervention and control groups at different time points throughout the intervention period. T-test analyses were conducted to compare differences in maternal oral health related attitudes and mothers' oral health outcomes at each assessment between intervention and control groups.

The differences with regard to changes over intervention time in the mean scores of maternal oral health related attitudes and their oral health outcomes between baseline (eight weeks) and 12 months were compared between intervention and control groups using t-tests. The use of differences in the mean scores allowed the analyses of all the data while excluding the two missing mothers at 12 months.

3. Results

A convenience sample of 36 Chinese newly arrived undocumented migrant mothers of new babies was recruited. One mother from the intervention group and one mother from the control group were lost to the 12-month follow-up as they moved from NI. The baseline information indicated that mothers' demographic characteristics were comparable between intervention and control group (Table 2).

Table 2. Demographic profiles of Chinese migrant families.

Demographic Profile	Intervention Group (n = 18)	Control Group (n = 18)	χ^2	p-Value
	Marital status			
single	1 (6%)	1 (6%)	0.00	1.00
married	17 (94%)	17 (94%)		
	Number of children			
1 child	6 (33%)	9 (50%)	0.72	0.31
More than 1 child	12 (67%)	9 (50%)		
	Baby gender			
female	8 (44%)	7 (39%)	0.11	0.76
male	10 (56%)	11 (61%)		
	Maternal education level (number of years)			
≤12 years	11 (61%)	9 (50%)	0.45	0.50
>12 years	7 (39%)	9 (50%)		
	Paternal education level (number of years)			
≤12 years	11 (61%)	8 (44%)	1.00	0.32
>12 years	7 (39%)	10 (56%)		
	Social deprivation level of residential area			
Deprived area (<220)	7 (39%)	10 (56%)	1.00	0.32
Less deprived area (≥221)	11 (61%)	8 (44%)		

3.1. Mothers' Oral Health Related Knowledge

At baseline, sixteen (44%) mothers irrespective of their groups correctly answered the question that they should start brushing baby's teeth as soon as the first teeth erupt. No other statistically significant difference was shown between intervention and control group mothers ($\chi^2 = 0.45$: $p = 0.50$).

At six-month assessment, of the 18 mothers who stated they had started brushing baby's teeth, a higher proportion of intervention group mothers (100%) knew that they should start brushing baby's teeth as soon as the first teeth erupted and the time they should start using fluoride toothpaste, compared with control group mothers (50%). However, there were no statistically significant differences between the two groups ($\chi^2 = 8.47$: $p = 0.11$). Sixteen intervention group mothers knew the right amount of fluoride toothpaste (i.e., "smear-size") when brushing their baby's teeth, as compared with control group mothers ($n = 2$).

At 12-month assessment, of the 20 mothers who stated they had started brushing baby's teeth, a statistically significant higher proportion of intervention group mothers (100%) knew that they should start brushing their baby's teeth and use fluoride toothpaste as soon as the first teeth erupted, compared with control group mothers (25%) ($\chi^2 = 14.12$: $p = 0.004$).

3.2. Mothers' Oral Health Related Attitudes

No statistically significant differences were shown in mothers' oral health related attitudes with regard to their intentions to brush baby's teeth and to control baby sugar consumption between intervention and control group mothers at baseline (Table 3).

Table 3. Comparison of maternal oral health related attitudes at baseline, 6 months, and 12 months between intervention and control group mothers.

Oral Health Related Attitudes	Intervention Group Mean Scores (95% CI)	Control Group Mean Scores (95% CI)	t	p-Value
Importance and intention to brush baby's teeth				
8 weeks	19.94 (19.02, 20.87)	19.61 (18.31, 20.91)	0.44	0.66
6 months	22.61 (21.56, 23.64)	18.83 (17.84, 19.83)	5.57	<0.001 ***
12 months	22.82 (21.93, 23.72)	18.76 (17.39, 20.14)	5.24	<0.001 ***
Importance and intention to control baby sugar snacking				
8 weeks	27.11 (25.64, 28.59)	27.94 (26.42, 2 9.47)	−0.83	0.41
6 months	31.11 (29.76, 32.46)	27.22 (25.91, 28.54)	4.35	<0.001 ***
12 months	32.59 (31.05, 34.13)	27.82 (26.13, 29.52)	4.40	<0.001 ***

95% CI: 95% Confidence Intervals. *** $p < 0.001$.

At six-month follow up, intervention group mothers had statistically significant higher mean attitudinal scores in "importance and intention to brush baby's teeth" and "importance and intention to control baby sugar snacking" compared with control group mothers (Table 3). Similar findings were shown in their 12-month follow-up assessment (Table 3).

When the changes of mothers' attitudinal mean scores over intervention period (eight weeks compared with 12 months) were measured, intervention group mothers had statistically significant changes in their perceived "importance and intention to brush baby's teeth" and "importance and intention to control baby sugar snacking" compared with control group mothers (Table 4). These changes in mothers' attitudinal mean scores between baseline (eight weeks), six months, and 12 months between intervention and control groups were also shown in line graphs (Figures 1 and 2).

Table 4. Comparison of changes in mean scores of maternal oral health knowledge and attitudinal scales by time between intervention and control groups.

Item	Group	8 Weeks Mean (95% CI)	12 Months Mean (95% CI)	Mean Change between Groups (Baseline vs. 12 months)	t	p-Value
Importance and intention to brush baby's teeth	Intervention	19.94 (19.02, 20.87)	22.82 (21.93, 23.72)	3.00 (1.56, 4.44)	3.79	0.001 **
	Control	19.61 (18.31, 20.91)	18.76 (17.39, 20.14)	−0.76 (−2.30, 0.77)		
Importance and intention to control baby sugar snacking	Intervention	27.11 (25.64, 28.59)	32.59 (31.05, 34.13)	5.76 (3.88, 7.65)	4.94	<0.001 ***
	Control	27.94 (26.42, 29.47)	27.82 (26.13, 29.52)	−0.18 (−1.89, 1.54)		

** $p < 0.01$, *** $p < 0.001$. 95% CI: 95% Confidence Intervals.

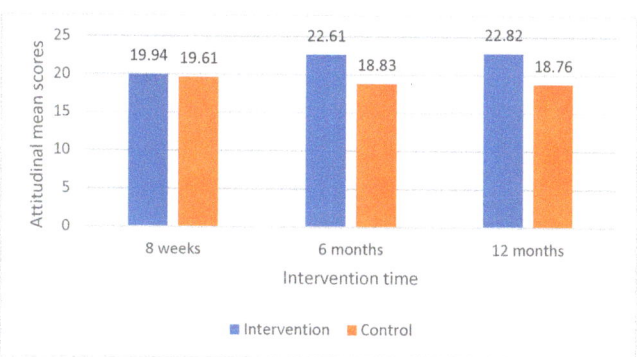

Figure 1. Changes in mean scores for importance and intention to brush baby's teeth for intervention and control groups.

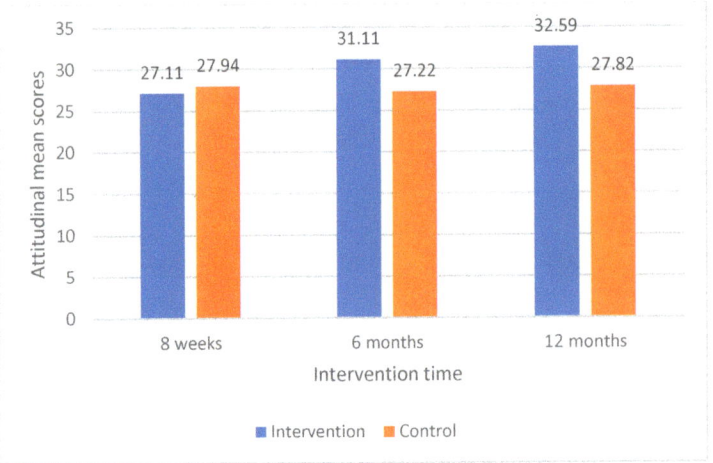

Figure 2. Changes in mean scores for importance and intention to control baby sugar snacking for intervention and control groups.

3.3. Mothers' Oral Health Related Behaviors

At baseline, twenty-eight (78%) mothers reported brushing their own teeth using fluoride toothpaste at least twice daily. No statistically significant difference was shown regarding reported daily frequencies of toothbrushing between intervention and control group mothers ($\chi^2 = 0.64$: $p = 0.42$). Twenty-three (64%) mothers stated they were registered with a dentist. Eight (22%) mothers stated that they attended for regular dental examinations and the remainder reported that they went to see a dentist either for treatment (6%) or only if having problem with their teeth or gums (47%). Nine (25%) mothers stated that they had never visited a dentist. No statistically significant differences were shown with regard to mothers' dental attendance at baseline.

At six-month assessment, 18 mothers (50%) stated that they had started brushing their baby's teeth at six months. Statistically significant higher proportions of intervention group mothers (89%) compared with control group mothers (11%) stated that they brushed their baby's teeth ($\chi^2 = 21.78$: $p < 0.001$). Statistically significant higher proportion of mothers from the intervention group compared with the control group stated that they brushed their own teeth at least twice a day ($\chi^2 = 5.78$: $p = 0.04$).

Twenty mothers (59%) reported that they brushed their baby's teeth at 12 months. Statistically significantly higher proportions of intervention group mothers (94%) stated that they brushed their baby's teeth ($p < 0.001$), compared with control group mothers (24%). No other statistical differences were found in mothers' other oral health related behaviors such as regular prevention oriented dental attendance.

3.4. Mothers' Obvious Decay Experience

There were no statistical significant differences in mothers' obvious decay experience (D_3MFT) between intervention and control group mothers at baseline ($t = 0.43$: $p = 0.67$), six months ($t = 0.40$: $p = 0.69$), and 12 months ($t = 0.10$: $p = 0.92$). No statistical significant difference in mothers' obvious decay experience (D_3MFT) over intervention period was found between intervention and control group mothers ($t = -1.05$: $p = 0.30$).

4. Discussion

The intervention has shown the promising effect in improving mothers' oral health related knowledge, perceived importance, and intention to take care of baby's teeth in terms of baby toothbrushing and sugar snacking, and their improved self-reported baby toothbrushing behaviors.

These findings have further addressed the importance of tailoring the community based oral health intervention through including the local community in the development of the intervention. More importantly, this intervention supports the proposition that health intervention for newly arrived migrant groups should be provided in a culturally appropriate manner using community health workers who speak the same language and share the same cultural background.

The recruited Chinese undocumented migrant mothers were characteristic of those with multiple social disadvantages: being undocumented migrants, had language difficulties, experienced problems in adapting the mainstream society, had lower levels of educational attainment, and resided in disadvantaged areas [28,29]. The limited literature suggested children of migrant families had poorer oral health compared with children of indigenous families [30]. A recent American study indicated a social pattern in children's regular dental visits with children of non-permanent residents having the lowest dental care utilization rate (32% had one or more dental visits in the last year), followed by children of permanent residents (41%), naturalized parents (50%), and US-born parents (>50%) [31]. To my knowledge, no other studies have concentrated on the oral health of undocumented migrant families living in the UK, therefore, this is the first study to report findings of oral health changes in terms of parental oral health related knowledge, attitudes, and behaviors after a community-based intervention delivered to this 'hard to reach' population.

Mothers in the intervention group of this study showed significant improvement in their oral health knowledge and self-reported behaviors in terms of controlling baby sugar consumption. Most of them knew that sugar was bad for teeth. It seemed that the intervention group mothers were ready to receive and assimilate this message about baby sugar snacking into their daily dietary regimens. Of interest was the finding that mothers in the intervention group reported significant improvement in their perceived importance and intervention to control baby sugar snacking. These are meaningful results as other studies have reported that prolonged bottle-feeding is found more often in migrant families [30,32]. Similar findings were reported in other parental oral health intervention programs for newly arrived migrant parents in terms of the effectiveness in improving parental oral health related knowledge, attitudes, and practices to take good care of children's teeth [33,34].

The other meaningful finding was the intervention group mothers had improved knowledge, perceived importance, and intention to brush baby's teeth, as well as their increased level of reported baby toothbrushing behaviors. These effects might be due to several reasons. First, mothers received culturally sensitive information of baby tooth decay and the importance of toothbrushing with fluoride toothpaste to prevent child tooth decay. Secondly, mothers were provided with a toothbrush and fluoride toothpaste for their infants and themselves. This meant that the financial costs and length of time adopting this healthy behavior was reduced, and thirdly, the young mothers were more responsive. It may be proposed that mothers were more ready to receive and act upon the oral health information about the welfare of their child. This was reflected in mothers being more likely to practice toothbrushing skills including establishing and assisting with child oral hygiene routines. In addition, it may be postulated that the adoption of parental toothbrushing could be thought of in terms of the developed trusting relationship with SY and adopted more "mainstream" lifestyle habits [35].

Despite the intervention group mothers' improved knowledge and attitudes towards baby toothbrushing, many mothers expressed frustrations when brushing their babies' teeth. For instance, some mothers complained that their babies would not sit quietly when having teeth brushed. These frustrations may affect mothers' confidence to develop and maintain routine oral hygiene practice. In other words, mothers who had low self-efficacy of baby toothbrushing might be less likely to adhere to this oral hygiene regimen, as suggested by the Health Action Process Approach [36]. Similar findings were reported by Marshman and her colleagues in terms of parents' perceived barriers to brushing children's teeth [37]. These included parental self-efficacy of toothbrushing and their beliefs about the consequences. It further indicated the importance of social support that may exhibit as an enabling factor to empower mothers to overcome such challenges for behavior change. This is particularly significant for undocumented migrant mothers whose home based routines might be chaotic. Therefore, it may be suggested that perhaps two home visits during the intervention period are not enough for Chinese undocumented migrant mothers to develop all aspects of parenting including child oral health home care. More intensive home visits would be recommended to encourage them to develop child rearing and parenting skills in a holistic approach that incorporates baby oral health related practice as a component.

While no statistically significant changes were found in mothers' obvious decay experience between intervention and control group mothers, this could be due to the relatively short period of the intervention to observe the changes in the clinical outcomes. The reason of including mothers' oral health status assessment in this intervention is according to the established strong association between mothers' active caries status and children's caries experience [16]. Future research should consider a longer follow-up period to record changes in parental oral health status as an indicator to evaluate the effect of parental oral health education interventions.

It may be suggested that this program has shown that giving oral health education to Chinese migrant mothers in a cultural sensitive manner using a one-to-one counselling strategy can assist in raising maternal awareness of child oral health during home visits. The role of SY must be considered as a factor with regard to the effectiveness of the intervention. SY, a Chinese mandarin speaker from mainland China, conducted the program. SY shares language, culture and lifestyle habits in common with Chinese migrant mothers living in Belfast. Moreover, SY was the same age as the mothers. Therefore SY understood the Chinese migrant mothers' psycho-social and health needs. The mothers, in turn, trusted her and consequently remained in the program. This partially explained the high retention rate in this study despite the small sample size. More importantly, this indicated the significance of the role of a community health worker sharing the same language and culture to understand and address the needs of this socially excluded group of mothers.

Limitation of the Study

There are several limitations in this study. The first is related to the sample. The sample gathered was a non-probability convenience sample. This is inevitable given this group is not recorded in the UK databases that could be used as sampling frames [38]. This is a most socially excluded group where the Chinese migrant population amounts to just a few thousand throughout Northern Ireland, therefore the limited sample we recruited was the entire population of accessible undocumented Chinese migrant mothers with babies aged less than eight weeks during the recruitment period. We acknowledge that the small size of the sample may increase the likelihood of type II error. Despite this concern, this work is innovative since there is little work done to promote oral health related knowledge, attitudes, and behaviors of this undocumented migrant group in Northern Ireland.

Secondly, as SY is the researcher and also the community health worker to implement the intervention, the present study did not use any blinding measures to reduce bias, which may affect the results of the study. Further, SY's high motivation may limit the reproductivity of similar findings for future interventions. However, this research work is regarded as meaningful for adding evidence into the limited literature to report effects of community-based interventions delivered to the undocumented migrant parents. Moreover, other studies have shown strong evidence in the effectiveness of having community health workers who share same language and culture to provide culturally appropriate health education [39].

Lastly, the oral health related behaviors regarding baby toothbrushing, mothers' own toothbrushing and regular dental attendance were self-reported by mothers who might have provided socially favorable answers. This may affect the reported effectiveness of this program. Furthermore, the evaluation of the program may have been contaminated by SY. Mothers in the control group asked SY for information regarding dental health and how to access health and social services. For ethical reasons, it was impossible not to have answered their requests. This concern of contamination allows a series of questions to be raised in relation to the effectiveness of the program. It would seem reasonable

5. Conclusions

To conclude, despite the small sample size of the present study, the community based parental oral health education program delivered in a culturally appropriate approach has shown promising effects to improve Chinese undocumented migrant mothers' knowledge, attitudes, and self-reported behaviors with a specific emphasis on baby toothbrushing and control of baby sugar consumption.

Funding: This research received no external funding.

Acknowledgments: I would like to acknowledge Anne Stevens for her kind support in conducting the dental examinations during the study. We would also like to thank the Chinese community leaders and all the Chinese mothers and babies for their kindest support in taking part of the Study.

Conflicts of Interest: The author declares no conflict of interest

References

1. Marcenes, W.; Kassebaum, N.J.; Bernabe, E.; Flaxman, A.; Naghavi, M.; Lopez, A.; Murray, C.J. Global burden of oral conditions in 1990–2010: A systematic analysis. *J. Dent. Res.* **2013**, *92*, 592–597. [CrossRef]
2. Paula, J.S.; Leite, I.C.; Almeida, A.B.; Ambrosano, G.M.; Pereira, A.C.; Mialhe, F.L. The influence of oral health conditions, socioeconomic status and home environment factors on schoolchildren's self-perception of quality of life. *Health Qual. Life Outcomes* **2012**, *10*, 6. [CrossRef]
3. Link, B.G.; Phelan, J. Social conditions as fundamental causes of disease. *J. Health Soc. Behav.* **1995**, 80–94. [CrossRef]
4. Phelan, J.C.; Link, B.G.; Tehranifar, P. Social conditions as fundamental causes of health inequalities: Theory, evidence, and policy implications. *J. Health Soc. Behav.* **2010**, *51*, S28–S40. [CrossRef]
5. Jackson, J.J. Race, national origin, ethnicity, and aging. In *Handbook of Aging and the Social Sciences*; Binstock, R.S., Ed.; Van Nostrand Reinhold: New York, NY, USA, 1985; pp. 264–303.
6. Assari, S.; Hani, N. Household Income and Children's Unmet Dental Care Need; Blacks' Diminished Return. *Dent. J.* **2018**, *6*, 17. [CrossRef] [PubMed]
7. Assari, S.; Thomas, A.; Caldwell, C.H.; Mincy, R.B. Blacks' Diminished Health Return of Family Structure and Socioeconomic Status; 15 Years of Follow-up of a National Urban Sample of Youth. *J. Urban Health* **2018**, *95*, 21–35. [CrossRef]
8. Assari, S. Parental Education Better Helps White than Black Families Escape Poverty: National Survey of Children's Health. *Economies* **2018**, *6*, 30. [CrossRef]
9. Assari, S. Unequal Gain of Equal Resources across Racial Groups. *Int. J. Health Policy Manag.* **2017**, *7*, 1–9. [CrossRef]
10. Riggs, E.; Gussy, M.; Gibbs, L.; van Gemert, C.; Waters, E.; Priest, N.; Watt, R.; Renzaho, A.M.; Kilpatrick, N. Assessing the cultural competence of oral health research conducted with migrant children. *Community Dent. Oral Epidemiol.* **2014**, *42*, 43–52. [CrossRef]
11. Gibbs, L.; de Silva, A.M.; Christian, B.; Gold, L.; Gussy, M.; Moore, L.; Calache, H.; Young, D.; Riggs, E.; Tadic, M.; et al. Child oral health in migrant families: A cross-sectional study of caries in 1–4 year old children from migrant backgrounds residing in Melbourne, Australia. *Community Dent. Health* **2016**, *33*, 100–106.
12. Kim Seow, W. Environmental, maternal, and child factors which contribute to early childhood caries: A unifying conceptual model. *Int. J. Paediatr. Dent.* **2012**, *22*, 157–168. [CrossRef] [PubMed]
13. Mattila, M.L.; Rautava, P.; Sillanpaa, M.; Paunio, P. Caries in five-year-old children and associations with family-related factors. *J. Dent. Res.* **2000**, *79*, 875–881. [CrossRef] [PubMed]
14. Vozza, I.; Capasso, F.; Marrese, E.; Polimeni, A.; Ottolenghi, L. Infant and Child Oral Health Risk Status Correlated to Behavioral Habits of Parents or Caregivers: A Survey in Central Italy. *J. Int. Soc. Prev. Community Dent.* **2017**, *7*, 95–99. [CrossRef] [PubMed]
15. Laitala, M.L.; Vehkalahti, M.M.; Virtanen, J.I. Frequent consumption of sugar-sweetened beverages and sweets starts at early age. *Acta Odontol. Scand.* **2018**, *76*, 105–110. [CrossRef] [PubMed]

16. Wan, A.K.; Seow, W.K.; Purdie, D.M.; Bird, P.S.; Walsh, L.J.; Tudehope, D.I. A longitudinal study of Streptococcus mutans colonization in infants after tooth eruption. *J. Dent. Res.* **2003**, *82*, 504–508. [CrossRef] [PubMed]
17. Wong, D.; Perez-Spiess, S.; Julliard, K. Attitudes of Chinese parents toward the oral health of their children with caries: A qualitative study. *Pediatr. Dent.* **2005**, *27*, 505–512. [PubMed]
18. Chu, C.H.; Chau, A.M.; Lo, E.C.; Lam, A. Planning and implementation of community oral health programs for caries management in children. *Gen. Dent.* **2012**, *60*, 210–215.
19. Mouradian, W.E.; Huebner, C.E.; Ramos-Gomez, F.; Slavkin, H.C. Beyond access: The role of family and community in children's oral health. *J. Dent. Educ.* **2007**, *71*, 619–631.
20. Glassman, P.; Harrington, M.; Namakian, M. Promoting oral health through community engagement. *J. Calif. Dent. Assoc.* **2014**, *42*, 465–470.
21. Ehmsen, B.K.; Biswas, D.; Jensen, N.K.; Krasnik, A.; Norredam, M. Undocumented migrants have diverse health problems. *Dan. Med. J.* **2014**, *61*, A4897.
22. Northern Ireland Statistics and Research Agency (NISAR). Northern Ireland Multiple Deprivation Measure 2005. Available online: http://www.nisra.gov.uk/archive/deprivation/NIMDM2005FullReport.pdf (accessed on 12 July 2006).
23. Services NIG. Available online: https://www.nidirect.gov.uk/articles/health-service-dental-charges-and-treatments (accessed on 18 November 2018).
24. Sadler, G.R.; Lee, H.-C.; Lim, R.S.-H.; Fullerton, J. Recruitment of hard-to-reach population subgroups via adaptations of the snowball sampling strategy. *Nurs. Health Sci.* **2010**, *12*, 369–374. [CrossRef] [PubMed]
25. Yuan, S.-Y.; Freeman, R. Can social support in the guise of an oral health education intervention promote mother–infant bonding in Chinese immigrant mothers and their infants? *Health Educ. J.* **2011**, *70*, 57–66. [CrossRef]
26. Adair, P.M.; Pine, C.M.; Burnside, G.; Nicoll, A.D.; Gillett, A.; Anwar, S.; Broukal, Z.; Chestnutt, I.G.; Declerck, D.; Ping, F.X.; et al. Familial and cultural perceptions and beliefs of oral hygiene and dietary practices among ethnically and socio-economicall diverse groups. *Community Dent. Health* **2004**, *21*, 102–111.
27. Pitts, N.B.; Evans, D.J.; Pine, C.M. British Association for the Study of Community Dentistry (BASCD) diagnostic criteria for caries prevalence surveys-1996/97. *Community Dent. Health* **1997**, *14* (Suppl. 1), 6–9.
28. Coulthard, M.; Walker, A.; Morgan, A. *People's Perceptions of Their Neighbourhood and Community Involvement: Results from the Social Capital Module of the General Household Survey 2000*; The Stationery Office: London, UK, 2002.
29. Moore, S.; Kawachi, I. Twenty years of social capital and health research: A glossary. *J. Epidemiol. Community Health* **2017**, *71*, 513–517. [CrossRef] [PubMed]
30. Woodward, G.L.; Leake, J.L.; Main, P.A. Oral health and family characteristics of children attending private or public dental clinics. *Community Dent. Oral Epidemiol.* **1996**, *24*, 253–259. [CrossRef] [PubMed]
31. Ziol-Guest, K.M.; Kalil, A. Health and medical care among the children of immigrants. *Child Dev.* **2012**, *83*, 1494–1500. [CrossRef]
32. Weinstein, P.; Smith, W.F.; Fraser-Lee, N.; Shimono, T.; Tsubouchi, J. Epidemiologic study of 19-month-old Edmonton, Alberta children: Caries rates and risk factors. *ASDC J. Dent. Child* **1996**, *63*, 426–433.
33. Brown, R.M.; Canham, D.; Cureton, V.Y. An oral health education program for Latino immigrant parents. *J. Sch. Nurs.* **2005**, *21*, 266–271. [CrossRef]
34. Harrison, R.L.; Wong, T. An oral health promotion program for an urban minority population of preschool children. *Community Dent. Oral Epidemiol.* **2003**, *31*, 392–399. [CrossRef]
35. Islam, M.K.; Merlo, J.; Kawachi, I.; Lindstrom, M.; Gerdtham, U.G. Social capital and health: Does egalitarianism matter? A literature review. *Int. J. Equity Health* **2006**, *5*, 3. [CrossRef] [PubMed]
36. Sniehotta, F.F.; Schwarzer, R.; Scholz, U.; Schüz, B. Action planning and coping planning for long-term lifestyle change: Theory and assessment. *Eur. J. Soc. Psychol.* **2005**, *35*, 565–576. [CrossRef]
37. Marshman, Z.; Ahern, S.M.; McEachan, R.R.C.; Rogers, H.J.; Gray-Burrows, K.A.; Day, P.F. Parents' Experiences of Toothbrushing with Children: A Qualitative Study. *JDR Clin. Trans. Res.* **2016**, *1*, 122–130. [CrossRef] [PubMed]

38. Newton, J.T.; Khan, F.A.; Bhavnani, V.; Pitt, J.; Gelbier, S.; Gibbons, D.E. Self-assessed oral health status of ethnic minority residents of South London. *Community Dent. Oral Epidemiol.* **2000**, *28*, 424–434. [CrossRef] [PubMed]
39. Andrews, J.O.; Felton, G.; Wewers, M.E.; Heath, J. Use of community health workers in research with ethnic minority women. *J. Nurs. Scholarsh.* **2004**, *36*, 358–365. [CrossRef] [PubMed]

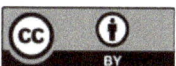

© 2019 by the author. Licensee MDPI, Basel, Switzerland. This article is an open access article distributed under the terms and conditions of the Creative Commons Attribution (CC BY) license (http://creativecommons.org/licenses/by/4.0/).

MDPI
St. Alban-Anlage 66
4052 Basel
Switzerland
Tel. +41 61 683 77 34
Fax +41 61 302 89 18
www.mdpi.com

Dentistry Journal Editorial Office
E-mail: dentistry@mdpi.com
www.mdpi.com/journal/dentistry

www.ingramcontent.com/pod-product-compliance
Lightning Source LLC
LaVergne TN
LVHW072000080526
838202LV00064B/6802